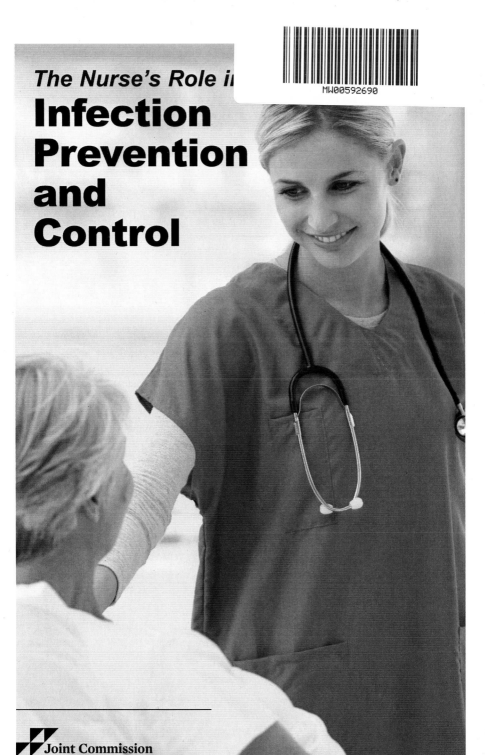

The Nurse's Role in
Infection Prevention and Control

▼▼ Joint Commission Resources

Project Manager: Andrew Bernotas
Editor and Manager, Publications: Victoria Gaudette
Associate Director, Production: Johanna Harris
Executive Director: Catherine Chopp Hinckley, Ph.D.
Joint Commission/JCR Reviewers: Diane Bell, Kelly Fugate, Cynthia Leslie, Virginia McCollum, and Susan Slavish

Joint Commission Resources Mission
The mission of Joint Commission Resources (JCR) is to continuously improve the safety and quality of health care in the United States and in the international community through the provision of education, publications, consultation, and evaluation services.

Joint Commission Resources educational programs and publications support, but are separate from, the accreditation activities of The Joint Commission. Attendees at Joint Commission Resources educational programs and purchasers of Joint Commission Resources publications receive no special consideration or treatment in, or confidential information about, the accreditation process.

The inclusion of an organization name, product, or service in a Joint Commission Resources publication should not be construed as an endorsement of such organization, product, or service, nor is failure to include an organization name, product, or service to be construed as disapproval.

This publication is designed to provide accurate and authoritative information in regard to the subject matter covered. Every attempt has been made to ensure accuracy at the time of publication; however, please note that laws, regulations, and standards are subject to change. Please also note that some of the examples in this publication are specific to the laws and regulations of the locality of the facility. The information and examples in this publication are provided with the understanding that the publisher is not engaged in providing medical, legal, or other professional advice. If any such assistance is desired, the services of a competent professional person should be sought.

Printed in the U.S.A. 5 4 3 2 1

Requests for permission to make copies of any part of this work should be mailed to
Permissions Editor
Department of Publications
Joint Commission Resources
One Renaissance Boulevard
Oakbrook Terrace, Illinois 60181 U.S.A.
permissions@jcrinc.com

ISBN: 978-1-59940-370-0
Library of Congress Control Number: 2009933650

For more information about Joint Commission Resources, please visit http://www.jcrinc.com.

Contents

Chapter 3. Partnering with Other Disciplines to Help Prevent and Control Infections

Chapter 4. The Nurse's Role in Educating Patients and Their Families on Safe Infection Prevention and Control Processes

Introduction

The Centers for Disease Control and Prevention estimates that each year, approximately 1.7 million patients admitted to acute care hospitals in the United States acquire infections that were not related to the condition for which they were hospitalized.[1] These infections result in close to 100,000 deaths and add between $4.5 to $5.7 billion per year to patient care costs.[1,2] Although the precise causes of health care–associated infections (HAIs) are difficult to identify, it has been estimated that approximately one third of HAIs could be prevented.[2]

Because of their proximity to patients and their pivotal role in health care delivery, nurses are in a unique position to participate in the development, implementation, and monitoring of infection prevention and control practices. In addition to following recommended infection prevention and control practices while providing direct patient care, nurses can also act as educators, role models, and patient advocates. They can serve on patient safety and infection prevention and control committees. Many may work as infection preventionists.

By incorporating infection prevention and control strategies into their everyday practices and by helping implement, monitor, and sustain infection prevention and control practices within health care organizations, nurses can play vital roles in the infection control process.

The Nurse's Role in Infection Prevention and Control examines the nurse's role in ensuring that patients, their families, other staff, and the public are protected from infections. It includes initiatives developed by other organizations that relate to specific topics and provides multiple examples of forms, handouts, checklists, and procedures. A detailed description of each chapter follows.

Chapter 1. Methods for Implementing and Sustaining Best Practices: What Nurses Can Do to Sustain Best Practices Every Day

This chapter discusses what nurses can do on an everyday basis to prevent and to control infections. It includes information about fostering a culture of safety, teaching others about infection prevention and control practices, serving as good examples to others, focusing on patient-centered care, and monitoring and reporting individual or systems failures. It also discusses opening the lines of communication with patients and families, evaluating health literacy, and obtaining a complete patient history.

Chapter 2. Educating Nursing Staff on Safe Infection Prevention and Control Practices

Before nurses can initiate infection prevention and control measures, they need to be properly educated. This chapter includes information about educating nursing staff regarding how to prevent and control infections while providing direct patient care, treatment, or services or preparing or administering medications. It also includes information about preventing cross-contamination when using charts and computers and about educating nursing staff in the following areas of infection control:

- Hand hygiene
- Surgical site infections (SSIs)
- Multidrug-resistant organisms (MDROs)
- Catheter-associated urinary tract infections (CAUTIs)
- Central line–associated bloodstream infections (CLABSIs)
- Ventilator-associated pneumonia (VAP)
- Influenza

Chapter 3. Partnering with Other Disciplines to Help Prevent and Control Infections

Effective infection prevention and control practices should be implemented by every member of the health care team. This chapter discusses how nurses can work with each other, as well as with physicians and infection preventionists, to prevent and to control infections. It also provides information about working with other patient care and nonclinical staff on infection prevention and control measures.

Chapter 4. The Nurse's Role in Educating Patients and Their Families on Safe Infection Prevention and Control Processes
This chapter discusses understanding patient and family needs beyond clinical components. It also includes information about cultural challenges to educational efforts, as well as instructions regarding how to conduct a lifestyle assessment and a home assessment. In addition, this chapter discusses patient education in the following areas:
- Standard precautions
- Contact, droplet, and airborne precautions
- Patient hygiene
- Supplies/equipment
- MDROs
- SSIs
- CAUTIs
- CLABSIs
- VAP
- Influenza
- Food safety
- Medications
- Pet safety
- Reporting concerns
- Discharge planning

Chapter 5. The Nurse's Role in Preventing and Controlling Infections in Special Settings and Populations
Infection prevention and control methods may differ based on the venue or patient population. This chapter discusses the nurse's role in preventing and controlling infections in home care, ambulatory care, surgery, emergency department, pediatrics, oncology, long term care, behavioral health care, maternity, and neonatal units.

Acknowledgments

Joint Commission Resources (JCR) gratefully acknowledges the time and insights of the following people and organizations:

- Sophie Harnage, R.N., B.S.N., clinical manager, Infusion Services, Sutter Roseville Medical Center, Roseville, CA
- Stephanie Holley, R.N., B.S.N., C.I.C., Quality Management Coordinator, Infection Control Professional and Nurse Epidemiologist, Program of Hospital Epidemiology, University of Iowa Hospitals and Clinics, Iowa City
- Cynthia Leslie, A.P.R.N., M.S.N., B.C., associate director, Standards Interpretation Group, The Joint Commission
- Pier Mania Mazza, Ospedale di Locarno, Switzerland
- Virginia McCollum, M.S.N., R.N., associate director, Standards Interpretation Group, The Joint Commission
- Mary McGoldrick, M.S., R.N., C.R.N.I., home care and hospice consultant, Home Health Systems, Inc., St. Simons Island, GA
- Jan Odom-Forren, R.N., M.S., C.P.A.N., F.A.A.N., perianesthesia and perioperative consultant and nursing instructor, University of Kentucky, Lexington
- Gail Potter-Bynoe, B.S., C.I.C., manager, Infection Prevention and Control, Children's Hospital Boston
- Beverly Robins, field director, Division of Accreditation and Certification Operations, The Joint Commission
- Susan Slavish, M.P.H., C.I.C., intermittent consultant for Joint Commission Resources and Joint Commission International
- Francine Westergaard, M.S.N., R.N., JCI/JCR consultant, Joint Commission International, Joint Commission Resources
- Laura Zitella, R.N., M.S., N.P., A.O.C.N., nurse practitioner, Division of Oncology, Stanford University Cancer Center, Stanford, CA

References

1. Centers for Disease Control and Prevention: *Estimates of Healthcare-Associated Infections.* Updated Jun. 15, 2009. http://www.cdc.gov/ncidod/dhqp/hai.html (accessed Mar. 25, 2009).
2. Joint Commission Resources: Health care–associated infections: Safeguards for infection-free care. *Source* 6:4–5,10, Feb. 2008.

Chapter 1
Methods for Implementing and Sustaining Best Practices
What Nurses Can Do to Sustain Best Practices Every Day

In many health care organizations, nurses provide the majority of direct patient care, so it is vital that they execute best practices for infection prevention and control. However, in addition to implementing infection prevention and control measures while providing direct patient care, nurses can use a number of methods to make sure that best practices are employed on a day-to-day basis to prevent and to control the transmission of infection. Some of those things may include systems changes, such as working to create a culture of safety. Others may be serving as examples to others or focusing on patient-centered care.

Creating a Culture of Safety

When nurses see systems problems that contribute to health care–associated infections (HAIs), they need to advocate for changes that will improve patient safety. One of the first steps in creating a safer health care environment is establishing a culture of safety. A safety culture flourishes when staff members feel comfortable reporting and discussing errors, when the organization actively works to learn from mistakes and to prevent future ones, and when safety is an organizational priority. Creating a culture of safety also involves moving away from blaming people for mistakes and toward identifying underlying system issues that can lead to errors.[1]

A safety culture is possible only when everyone in an organization is committed to proactive error prevention and safety improvement efforts. Effective communication between staff and licensed independent practitioners (LIPs), leadership, and patients and their families is essential.[1]

Staff members and LIPs within an organization have different backgrounds, beliefs, values, education, and experience. Diversity can help an organization develop a multifaceted perspective on issues, but it can also lead to confusion and misunderstanding. That is why it is vital for leaders to create and to promote a common values system that supports patient safety.[1]

Typically, the leaders develop and communicate the organization's mission, vision, and values to staff members as well as those served by the organization. Part of the planning process includes developing an organizationwide safety program that integrates all patient safety activities.[1]

Leaders are responsible for fostering a safe environment, including the following[1]:
• Establishing processes for recognition and acknowledgement of risks
• Initiating actions to reduce risks
• Creating internal reporting mechanisms
• Focusing on systems critical to the safety and quality of care, treatment, and services
• Minimizing blame and retribution
• Encouraging organizational learning about errors
• Supporting sharing of knowledge
• Establishing a "just culture" (a culture where health care workers feel comfortable disclosing errors—including their own—while maintaining professional accountability)

Leaders must implement an integrated patient safety program in the organization. This involves establishing procedures for immediately responding to system or process failures, including care, treatment, or services to the affected individual(s); containing risk to others; and preserving factual information for subsequent analysis. Clear systems for internal and external reporting of information about system or process failures must be present. Also, defined responses to various types of unanticipated adverse events must be clear. Additionally, processes for conducting proactive risk-assessment and risk-reduction activities must be in place.[1]

Measuring Your Organization's Safety Culture

Creating behavioral norms around safety is often accomplished when an organization's leaders establish a strategic direction where patient safety is regarded as a priority around which the efforts of the entire organization must be focused. The extent to which patient safety is a strategic priority may reflect the attitudes of leadership toward patient safety, but it may not reflect the organization's culture. Measuring an organization's culture of safety may be based on subjective assessments through staff questionnaires that measure staff's willingness to report errors and the organization's prioritization of increased safety through interventions. Survey tools are available to help assess the safety culture among staff in an organization (*see* Figure 1-1, pages 4–7). Some organizations that have conducted employee surveys have found a disparity between the perceptions of organization leadership and other staff members with regard to a culture of safety.[1]

Changing the Culture

A culture of safety focuses on four fundamental elements[1]:

- Developing a sense of trust among all stakeholders and caregivers
- Disseminating information to all levels of managers and employees and ensuring that the message is communicated
- Developing and supporting a proactive approach instead of a reactive approach
- Ensuring a sincere commitment to a culture that places safety as the first priority

Creating a culture of safety involves developing norms and values that assure patient safety and quality outcomes by managing relationships among and between physicians, nurses, and allied health professionals. It also means developing expectations for which each individual, each department, each patient care team, and each administrator will be held accountable.[1]

According to the Institute for Healthcare Improvement,[2] some organizations are now adopting language that can be used to interrupt an error as it is occurring in practice. An example may be a phrase, such as, "I need a little clarity here" when one clinician witnesses a potential error.[2] When this phrase is used, the practicing clinician knows to stop and listen. The communication should be clear and respectful, and it should not alarm the patient.[2]

If no such system is in place, the person witnessing the potential error should speak to the clinician or other staff member directly.[2] Again, the communication should be clear and respectful, and the person being confronted should not respond in a defensive manner.[2]

Monitoring and Reporting Individual or System Failures

Nurses should feel comfortable reporting errors that lead to HAIs, even when the errors are their own. In a culture of safety and quality, all individuals will accept

Figure 1-1. Hospital Survey on Patient Safety Culture

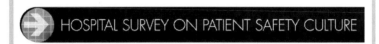

HOSPITAL SURVEY ON PATIENT SAFETY CULTURE

INSTRUCTIONS

This survey asks for your opinions about patient safety issues, medical error, and event reporting in your hospital and will take about 10 to 15 minutes to complete.

- An *"event"* is defined as any type of error, mistake, incident, accident, or deviation, regardless of whether or not it results in patient harm.

- *"Patient safety"* is defined as the avoidance and prevention of patient injuries or adverse events resulting from the processes of health care delivery.

SECTION A: Your Work Area/Unit

In this survey, think of your "unit" as the work area, department, or clinical area of the hospital where you spend *most* of your work time or provide *most* of your clinical services.

What is your primary work area or unit in this hospital? Mark ONE answer by filling in the circle.

○ a. Many different hospital units/No specific unit

○ b. Medicine (non-surgical)
○ c. Surgery
○ d. Obstetrics
○ e. Pediatrics
○ f. Emergency department

○ g. Intensive care unit (any type)
○ h. Psychiatry/mental health
○ i. Rehabilitation
○ j. Pharmacy
○ k. Laboratory

○ l. Radiology
○ m. Anesthesiology
○ n. Other, please specify:

Please indicate your agreement or disagreement with the following statements about your work area/unit. Mark your answer by filling in the circle.

Think about your hospital work area/unit...	Strongly Disagree	Disagree	Neither	Agree	Strongly Agree
1. People support one another in this unit	①	②	③	④	⑤
2. We have enough staff to handle the workload	①	②	③	④	⑤
3. When a lot of work needs to be done quickly, we work together as a team to get the work done	①	②	③	④	⑤
4. In this unit, people treat each other with respect	①	②	③	④	⑤
5. Staff in this unit work longer hours than is best for patient care	①	②	③	④	⑤
6. We are actively doing things to improve patient safety	①	②	③	④	⑤
7. We use more agency/temporary staff than is best for patient care	①	②	③	④	⑤
8. Staff feel like their mistakes are held against them	①	②	③	④	⑤
9. Mistakes have led to positive changes here	①	②	③	④	⑤
10. It is just by chance that more serious mistakes don't happen around here	①	②	③	④	⑤
11. When one area in this unit gets really busy, others help out	①	②	③	④	⑤
12. When an event is reported, it feels like the person is being written up, not the problem	①	②	③	④	⑤

1

(continued)

Figure 1-1. Hospital Survey on Patient Safety Culture, *continued*

SECTION A: Your Work Area/Unit (continued)

Think about your hospital work area/unit...

	Strongly Disagree	Disagree	Neither	Agree	Strongly Agree
13. After we make changes to improve patient safety, we evaluate their effectiveness	①	②	③	④	⑤
14. We work in "crisis mode" trying to do too much, too quickly	①	②	③	④	⑤
15. Patient safety is never sacrificed to get more work done	①	②	③	④	⑤
16. Staff worry that mistakes they make are kept in their personnel file	①	②	③	④	⑤
17. We have patient safety problems in this unit	①	②	③	④	⑤
18. Our procedures and systems are good at preventing errors from happening	①	②	③	④	⑤

SECTION B: Your Supervisor/Manager

Please indicate your agreement or disagreement with the following statements about your immediate supervisor/manager or person to whom you directly report. Mark your answer by filling in the circle.

	Strongly Disagree	Disagree	Neither	Agree	Strongly Agree
1. My supervisor/manager says a good word when he/she sees a job done according to established patient safety procedures	①	②	③	④	⑤
2. My supervisor/manager seriously considers staff suggestions for improving patient safety	①	②	③	④	⑤
3. Whenever pressure builds up, my supervisor/manager wants us to work faster, even if it means taking shortcuts	①	②	③	④	⑤
4. My supervisor/manager overlooks patient safety problems that happen over and over	①	②	③	④	⑤

SECTION C: Communications

How often do the following things happen in your work area/unit? Mark your answer by filling in the circle.

Think about your hospital work area/unit...

	Never	Rarely	Some-times	Most of the time	Always
1. We are given feedback about changes put into place based on event reports	①	②	③	④	⑤
2. Staff will freely speak up if they see something that may negatively affect patient care	①	②	③	④	⑤
3. We are informed about errors that happen in this unit	①	②	③	④	⑤
4. Staff feel free to question the decisions or actions of those with more authority	①	②	③	④	⑤
5. In this unit, we discuss ways to prevent errors from happening again	①	②	③	④	⑤
6. Staff are afraid to ask questions when something does not seem right	①	②	③	④	⑤

2

(continued)

Figure 1-1. Hospital Survey on Patient Safety Culture, *continued*

SECTION D: Frequency of Events Reported

In your hospital work area/unit, when the following mistakes happen, *how often are they reported?* Mark your answer by filling in the circle.

	Never	Rarely	Some-times	Most of the time	Always
1. When a mistake is made, but is *caught and corrected before affecting the patient*, how often is this reported?	①	②	③	④	⑤
2. When a mistake is made, but has *no potential to harm the patient*, how often is this reported?	①	②	③	④	⑤
3. When a mistake is made that *could harm the patient*, but does not, how often is this reported?	①	②	③	④	⑤

SECTION E: Patient Safety Grade

Please give your work area/unit in this hospital an overall grade on patient safety. Mark ONE answer.

○	○	○	○	○
A	**B**	**C**	**D**	**E**
Excellent	Very Good	Acceptable	Poor	Failing

SECTION F: Your Hospital

Please indicate your agreement or disagreement with the following statements about your hospital. Mark your answer by filling in the circle.

Think about your hospital...	Strongly Disagree	Disagree	Neither	Agree	Strongly Agree
1. Hospital management provides a work climate that promotes patient safety...	①	②	③	④	⑤
2. Hospital units do not coordinate well with each other	①	②	③	④	⑤
3. Things "fall between the cracks" when transferring patients from one unit to another...	①	②	③	④	⑤
4. There is good cooperation among hospital units that need to work together	①	②	③	④	⑤
5. Important patient care information is often lost during shift changes	①	②	③	④	⑤
6. It is often unpleasant to work with staff from other hospital units .	①	②	③	④	⑤
7. Problems often occur in the exchange of information across hospital units	①	②	③	④	⑤
8. The actions of hospital management show that patient safety is a top priority...	①	②	③	④	⑤
9. Hospital management seems interested in patient safety only after an adverse event happens	①	②	③	④	⑤
10. Hospital units work well together to provide the best care for patients...	①	②	③	④	⑤
11. Shift changes are problematic for patients in this hospital...........	①	②	③	④	⑤

SECTION G: Number of Events Reported

In the past 12 months, how many event reports have you filled out and submitted? Mark ONE answer.

- ○ a. No event reports
- ○ b. 1 to 2 event reports
- ○ c. 3 to 5 event reports
- ○ d. 6 to 10 event reports
- ○ e. 11 to 20 event reports
- ○ f. 21 event reports or more

3

(continued)

Figure 1-1. Hospital Survey on Patient Safety Culture, *continued*

SECTION H: Background Information
This information will help in the analysis of the survey results. **Mark ONE answer by filling in the circle.**

1. How long have you worked in this hospital?

   ○ a. Less than 1 year   ○ d. 11 to 15 years
   ○ b. 1 to 5 years   ○ e. 16 to 20 years
   ○ c. 6 to 10 years   ○ f. 21 years or more

2. How long have you worked in your current hospital work area/unit?

   ○ a. Less than 1 year   ○ d. 11 to 15 years
   ○ b. 1 to 5 years   ○ e. 16 to 20 years
   ○ c. 6 to 10 years   ○ f. 21 years or more

3. Typically, how many hours per week do you work in this hospital?

   ○ a. Less than 20 hours per week   ○ d. 60 to 79 hours per week
   ○ b. 20 to 39 hours per week   ○ e. 80 to 99 hours per week
   ○ c. 40 to 59 hours per week   ○ f. 100 hours per week or more

4. What is your staff position in this hospital? Mark ONE answer that best describes your staff position.

   ○ a. Registered Nurse   ○ h. Dietician
   ○ b. Physician Assistant/Nurse Practitioner   ○ i. Unit Assistant/Clerk/Secretary
   ○ c. LVN/LPN   ○ j. Respiratory Therapist
   ○ d. Patient Care Assistant/Hospital Aide/Care Partner   ○ k. Physical, Occupational, or Speech Therapist
   ○ e. Attending/Staff Physician   ○ l. Technician (e.g., EKG, Lab, Radiology)
   ○ f. Resident Physician/Physician in Training   ○ m. Administration/Management
   ○ g. Pharmacist   ○ n. Other, please specify:

5. In your staff position, do you typically have direct interaction or contact with patients?

   ○ a. YES, I typically have direct interaction or contact with patients.
   ○ b. NO, I typically do NOT have direct interaction or contact with patients.

6. How long have you worked in your current specialty or profession?

   ○ a. Less than 1 year   ○ d. 11 to 15 years
   ○ b. 1 to 5 years   ○ e. 16 to 20 years
   ○ c. 6 to 10 years   ○ f. 21 years or more

SECTION I: Your Comments
Please feel free to write any comments about patient safety, error, or event reporting in your hospital.

THANK YOU FOR COMPLETING THIS SURVEY.

4

This survey tool can be used to assess staff opinion regarding safety issues.

Source: Agency for Healthcare Research and Quality.

What Would You Do?

You are in a patient room while a surgeon is making rounds. You see the physician put on gloves and then inspect a patient's wound. When he is finished, he does not remove the gloves or perform hand hygiene. Instead, he goes over to inspect the wound of the person in the next bed. What would you do?

In this scenario, infections could be spread from one patient's wound to another via the physician's hands. Because it is the nurse's responsibility to protect the patient, it is essential that he or she stop the physician from touching the other patient with soiled hands. The nurse might say something like, "Doctor, can I see you outside for just a moment?" When the nurse gets the doctor outside the room, he or she might say, "I know you are busy and it was probably just an oversight, but I noticed that you forgot to remove your gloves and perform hand hygiene between patients. I am concerned that the patient in the second bed might be susceptible to infection."

This statement gives the physician the opportunity to correct a potential error without feeling as though he is being blamed. Allowing that the potential error could have been an oversight due to a busy schedule may also keep the physician from becoming defensive.

that safety and quality of patient care, treatment, and services is a personal responsibility, and they will work together to minimize any harm that might result from unsafe or poor quality care. Teamwork, open discussions of concerns about safety, and internal and external reporting of safety and quality issues are encouraged.[3] This type of culture flourishes when staff members feel comfortable reporting and discussing errors, when the organization actively works to learn from mistakes and to prevent future ones, and when safety is an organizational priority.[1]

A reporting culture is one in which patients and staff readily report all errors and near misses to allow staff members to learn from the experiences.[1] Creating a reporting culture involves moving away from blaming people for mistakes and toward identifying underlying system issues that can lead to HAIs.[1] A reporting culture is not meant to be antagonistic; the ultimate goal is to improve processes and outcomes.

A reporting culture is possible only when everyone in an organization is committed to proactive error prevention and safety improvement efforts. Effective communication between staff, leadership, and patients (and their families) is essential.[1] The following are strategies to support and to improve a reporting culture[1]:

- Develop a documentation system that is easy to use.
- Develop a reporting system that focuses on knowledge sharing.
- Provide feedback to staff on all issues reported.
- Develop measures of success (for example, increased number of reports).
- Prioritize improvement initiatives based on themes discovered and potential risks revealed.

Opening the Lines of Communication with Patients and Families

Each nurse-patient encounter is an opportunity for both parties to communicate—that is, to speak, to listen, to understand, and to respond appropriately to what the other has just said. Communication is the foundation for developing rapport and partnership. It is essential to patient satisfaction and patient safety. Yet, on average, clinicians listen to their patients for 18 to 23 seconds before interrupting.[4] The act of interrupting accomplishes at least three things: (1) it stops the flow of information, increasing the chances the clinician will miss something important that the patient would have revealed if allowed a little more time to speak; (2) it increases the likelihood of the patient ending the clinical interview with the phrase, "Oh, by the way," also known as the "doorknob question"; and (3) it stops the two-way communication that a relationship needs to develop.[4]

Because people have different styles of communication, the strategies nurses should use to communicate effectively with their patients will differ from one patient to another. Nurses may need to let some patients speak until they are finished, gently guide others who tend to ramble to focus on their main problems, or question and read the patients' body language to elicit information when none is forthcoming.[4]

Patients will be more comfortable sharing their personal and medical histories and other potentially important information if they feel at ease with their nurses.

Patients are put at ease when nurses convey warmth, understanding, and confidence in their patients and when they let patients know that their participation in their care is welcome and invited. All the information that the patient discusses—whether related to symptoms, medical history, potential adverse reactions to medication, or concerns about the potential for medical errors—is potentially important. Nurses can put patients at ease by letting them know that no question is too trivial and no piece of information is too minor to share.[4]

Empowering the Patient and Family to Speak Up!

In March 2002, The Joint Commission, together with the Centers for Medicare & Medicaid Services, launched a national campaign to urge patients to take roles in preventing health care errors by becoming active, involved, and informed participants on the health care team. The program features brochures, posters, and buttons on a variety of patient safety topics. In a survey conducted in 2008, more than 1,900 organizations responded that the Speak Up™ program has promoted and increased communication with patients and staff about safety. Speak Up encourages the public to:

Speak up if you have questions or concerns, and if you do not understand, ask again. It is your body, and you have a right to know.

Pay attention to the care you are receiving. Make sure you are getting the right treatments and medications from the right health care professionals. Do not assume anything.

Educate yourself about your diagnosis, the medical tests you are undergoing, and your treatment plan.

Ask a trusted family member or friend to be your advocate.

Know what medications you take and why you take them. Medication errors are the most common health care mistakes.

Use a hospital, clinic, surgery center, or other type of health care organization that has undergone a rigorous on-site evaluation against established state-of-the-art quality and safety standards, such as that provided by The Joint Commission.

Participate in all decisions about your treatment. You are the center of the health care team.

All Speak Up materials are available at http://www.jointcommission.org/PatientSafety/SpeakUp. Additional resources from the Joint Commission can also be found on Web sites such as Facebook, You Tube, and Twitter.

Sidebar 1-1.

Five Things Patients and Families Can Do to Prevent Infection

The Speak Up initiative advises patients and families to do the following five things to help prevent infection:

1. Clean your hands.
2. Make sure health care providers clean their hands or wear gloves.
3. Cover your mouth and nose (when sneezing or coughing).
4. If you are sick, avoid close contact with others.
5. Get shots to avoid disease and to fight the spread of infection.

Evaluating Health Literacy

Health literacy is the ability to read, to understand, and to effectively use basic medical instructions and information. Low health literacy can affect anyone of any age, ethnicity, background, or education level.[5]

According to the Partnership for Clear Health Communication, people with low health literacy do the following[5]:

- Are often less likely to adhere to prescribed treatment and self-care regimens
- Fail to seek preventive care and are at higher (more than double) risk for hospitalization
- Remain in the hospital nearly two days longer than adults with higher health literacy
- Often require additional care that results in annual health care costs that are four times higher than for those with higher literacy skills

The total number of people in the United States who have limited health literacy is more than 89 million.[6] Health literacy issues and ineffective communication place patients at greater risk of preventable adverse events. If a patient does not understand the implications of her or his diagnosis and the importance of prevention and treatment plans or cannot access health care services because of communication problems, an untoward event may occur. The same is true if the patient's health care providers do not understand the patient or the cultural context within which the patient receives critical information. Cultural, language, and communication barriers—together or alone—have great potential to lead to mutual misunderstandings between patients and their nurses.[1]

A common cause of patients' misunderstandings may be a failure to communicate on both sides. On the one hand, nurses often fail to realize that not all patients do the following:

• Understand medical jargon
• Have reading skills that allow them to read or to understand forms on their own
• Understand the oral explanations their nurses provide
• Really understand what they have agreed to when they sign consent forms

On the other hand, patients may fail to tell their nurses that they do not understand what they have read or heard, may not ask for help to interpret the required forms, and may not always ask questions that would let nurses know that further explanation is needed. If the cause of a patient's misunderstanding is the failure to communicate clearly and completely on both sides, then the solution must involve both sides. Because nurses have more authority to manage communication within the nurse-patient relationship, it is up to nurses not only to communicate more clearly and simply with all patients but to recognize that some patients need more, or different, types of communication to aid their understanding[4] (*see* Sidebar 1-2, page 13, for tips on improving effective communication). Nurses literally have to understand where their patients "are coming from"—the beliefs, values, and cultural mores and traditions that influence how health care information is shared and received.[7] Additionally, they need to be careful to also consider the patient as an individual rather than merely generalizing.

For people with low literacy skills, navigating the health system can be a nightmare. Deciphering hospital signage—"cardiac catheterization laboratory and outpatient radiology this way"—completing complex forms; interacting with health care providers; following medication instructions; and coping with real or perceived slights from hospital personnel place high demands on those with low literacy skills.[7]

Health care organization leaders are responsible for creating and maintaining cultures of quality and safety. This includes ensuring that nurses and other staff members communicate with patients on levels that the patients can understand. Yet awareness of the prevalence of health literacy issues is low among health care executives and other managers.[1]

Sidebar 1-2. Tips for Improving Effective Communication

The following tips can help your organization improve communications between staff and patients[1]:

- Raise awareness throughout the organization of the impact of health literacy and English proficiency on patient safety.
- Educate all staff in the organization to recognize and to respond appropriately to patients with literacy and language challenges.
- Create patient-centered environments that stress the use of clear communication in all interactions with patients, from the reception desk to discharge planning.
- Modify strategies for compliance with The Joint Commission's National Patient Safety Goals to accommodate patients with special literacy and language needs.
- Hire well-trained medical interpreters for patients with low English proficiency or who are deaf.
- Create organization cultures of safety and quality that value patient-centered communication as an integral component of delivering patient-centered care.

Nurses should know and reflect the communities they serve, including knowledge of patient demographics, such as age, family size, religion, and socioeconomic status. In addition, nurses should know the primary ethnic groups and languages through which their patients express themselves and the general literacy level of the community.[1] They should also be aware of any community-related public health concerns that might lead to the spread of infection.

Testing Comprehension Levels and Understanding

Health literacy plays a major role in whether a patient understands his or her diagnosis, how care instructions are interpreted, and whether the patient follows instructions. How can nurses tell who understands them and who does not, who has low literacy skills and who does not, and who would benefit if a nurse used a different approach to communicating? It may be difficult to tell from outward appearances which patients have low literacy skills and which do not. Most patients with low literacy skills are white, native-born Americans; many are from ethnic and racial minorities.[4] People with low literacy skills tend to be poor, less educated, and elderly, with physical and mental disabilities as well as multiple health problems.[4] But demographic information does not necessarily tell the whole story.

It is important that nurses learn to recognize the behaviors of patients with low health literacy skills. This may not be so easy, because many patients tend to be good at covering up their deficiencies, according to literacy advocate Toni Cordell.[4] When a patient says, "I left my reading glasses at home. Can you read this to me?" nurses should dig deeper and assess the patient's health literacy skills. Other behaviors, including the following, might also indicate a literacy problem[5,6]:

- Registration forms are incomplete or inaccurately completed.
- Appointments are frequently missed.
- The patient avoids situations that require him or her to read.
- The patient does not comply with medication regimens.
- The patient does not ask questions.
- Appointments for laboratory tests, imaging tests, or referrals to consultants are not scheduled or are missed.
- The patient requests to bring written documents home to discuss with a spouse or child.
- The patient complains of a headache or other health problem too severe to allow reading.
- The patient cannot restate information received in his or her own words.

If the nurse discovers that a patient does have low health literacy, he or she can do a number of things to assist. These may include helping the patient read or fill out forms; not using medical jargon; speaking slowly, especially when giving instructions; using the teach-back method; writing simple instructions; and using pictographs or videos.[8]

Obtaining a Complete Patient History

Obtaining a complete patient history helps the nurse understand not only the patient's biological health issues but also any social, emotional, cultural, or spiritual issues that may affect the patient's care.[9] A complete health history includes the following six components[9]:

1. **Biographical data.** This includes the patient's name, address, date of birth, place of birth, marital status, occupation, type of insurance, and social history.

2. **Chief complaint.** Why has the patient sought medical treatment?
3. **History of present illness.** When did the illness begin? Has it gotten worse over time? What has the patient tried so far?
4. **Health history.** The health history includes a review of past or chronic medical problems; previous injuries or surgeries; current medications (including over-the-counter medications or herbal supplements); and allergies to food, medications, or latex. This is also a good time to inquire about immunizations and recent exposure to or history of communicable diseases, such as measles, mumps, rubella, chicken pox, diphtheria, rheumatic fever, streptococcal infections, tuberculosis, sexually transmitted diseases, or HIV/AIDS. Risk factors for other types of infections, such as recent hospitalization, living in a group home, or traveling abroad, should also be assessed.
5. **Family history.** When inquiring about family history, the nurse should ask about the health status of close relatives who are still living and the cause of death for those who are not. This may include a history of heart disease, cancer, stroke, diabetes, hypertension, or high cholesterol. It may also include a history of communicable diseases, such as tuberculosis or methicillin-resistant *Staphylococcus aureus.*
6. **Lifestyle assessment.** The lifestyle assessment includes gathering information about lifestyle issues that may affect a patient's treatment and recovery, such as smoking, poor nutritional intake or overeating, substance abuse, or poor hygiene practices. For more information about lifestyle issues, see Chapter 4.

Nurses can use a number of communication strategies to elicit information from the patient when obtaining a patient history. For more information about communication strategies, see Chapter 4.

Teaching Others About Infection Prevention and Control Practices

A large part of what nurses do on a daily basis involves teaching. Not only are nurses responsible for the majority of patient education, they are also responsible for teaching others about infection prevention and control. Certified nursing assistants, patient care technicians, and nursing students all work closely with nurses and look to them to provide education and instruction. However, nurses can also be involved in teaching infection prevention and control practices to other clinical and nonclinical personnel.

Although this role is primarily that of an infection preventionist, nurses frequently also serve on organizational infection prevention and control committees, where they may review the literature for evidence-based practices to help prevent and control the transmission of infection. In this role, a nurse may bring best practices to the committee's attention and work with the infection preventionist to develop new protocols for infection prevention and control. In this capacity, the nurse may be partially responsible for the development of new policies that will be used by all clinical staff, including physicians. The nurse may also be responsible for staff education at in-services or nursing staff or medical staff meetings, or for developing educational materials.

For nonclinical staff, the nurse may work with the infection preventionist to help teach courses in hand hygiene or about isolation precautions. Also working collaboratively with the infection preventionist, the nurse may assist with or lead courses for environmental services staff about how to prevent the transmission of multidrug-resistant organisms.

Nurses are frequently asked questions by friends, family, and neighbors, which may lead to opportunities to educate members of the community about infection prevention and control practices.

For more information about nurses partnering with other disciplines to prevent or to control infection, see Chapter 3.

Nurses Serving as Examples to Others

For patients, nursing assistants, and nursing students, nurses are often looked upon as role models. Therefore, it is important that they consistently use best practices. It is one thing to educate others about infection prevention and control measures, but those educational efforts will have been in vain if those on the receiving end observe the instructor ignoring his or her own instructions.

Nurses can serve as examples to patients and other staff members not only by instructing them about appropriate infection prevention and control techniques but also by strictly adhering to infection prevention and control policies. This may include allowing others to see them perform hand hygiene between patients, donning gown and gloves before entering the room of a patient on contact precautions, using aseptic technique when inserting urinary catheters, raising the head of the bed for a patient who is on a ventilator, or not coming to work when ill.

Focusing on Patient-Centered Care

The nurse should act as the patient's advocate 100% of the time. Patient advocates (also known as patient representatives or patient ombudsmen) further the goals, needs, and preferences of the person for whom they are advocating. "The patient advocate has a challenging role: being the voice for another person," says Laura Weil, director of the Patient Representative Department of Beth Israel Medical Center, New York, and a faculty member in the Health Advocacy Graduate program at Sarah Lawrence College.[10]

Patient advocacy is at the heart of patient-centered care—a strategy that encourages the patient and family to participate in the care by speaking up and asking questions. It is one part of a systemwide, collaborative effort to create optimal outcomes for clinicians, patients, and families.[10]

"When you talk about advocating," says Gerald Hickson, M.D., associate dean for Clinical Affairs and director of the Center for Patient and Professional Advocacy at Vanderbilt University Medical Center, Nashville, Tennessee, "it can be as trivial as 'my room temperature is wrong' to 'I'm having a serious complication and nobody will listen.'" For patient advocacy to work, nurses constantly need to review what is going on by doing such things as asking the patient or family members if they have any concerns or monitoring the hand-hygiene practices of the patient and/or other staff members. Constant review and intervention is one way to implement patient advocacy as a patient-safety strategy.[10]

"Through collaboration with our learning center, nursing leadership, patient advocacy office, and center for patient and professional advocacy, we've created policies to promote centralization of complaints and provide better service recovery," Hickson says.

Some organizations directly involve the patient and families. "Recognizing and utilizing the special knowledge of the patient's loved ones is an important element of patient safety," Weil says. Beth Israel is testing a policy of allowing families to initiate a rapid response team. "Our new program enables a family member to independently access a team of specially trained doctors and nurses for immediate intervention," Weil says.[10]

In addition to establishing ombudsman departments, integrating patient representatives on units, and training all health care workers to advocate for the patient, some organizations use patient education videos to encourage advocacy and patient safety. At Vanderbilt, for example, patients and their family members watch a video inviting them to help the staff with several safety goals (for example, helping clinicians remember to wash their hands and to check patient identifications before taking blood or giving medications).[10]

Nurses can use the following strategies to help them serve as patient advocates[10]:

1. **Educate the patient.** Avoiding medical jargon, explain the patient's health situation and options for care in easy-to-understand language. Have the patient repeat it back to you to ensure understanding. This is an important tool to help determine whether the patient has sufficient information to make decisions about his or her health care.

2. **Help the patient define his or her treatment goals by listening carefully and encouraging the patient to voice his or her opinions.** The clinician, family, and patient may have different goals. As part of the process of clarifying goals, the patient advocate must be mindful of his or her own value system and biases. An advocate also has the difficult job of being honest when the patient's expectations may be unrealistic.

3. **Communicate with the patient's other caregivers and encourage them to do the right thing for the patient.** Communication among caregivers and patients means asking questions and facilitating discussion in a cooperative, respectful way. Two key concepts are:
   a. Optimism ("We will find a way to talk about this effectively.")
   b. Acknowledgement of common ground ("We all want what's best for the patient.")
   For example, saying "It would really be helpful to me if you could take a few minutes to explain the choices we're facing" reflects the above concepts much better than saying, "I've been waiting all day for you to tell me what's going on." Using *we* helps engage everyone in the same collaborative process.

4. **Ensure that care is provided in the safest manner possible.** "Advocacy includes reviewing when things *don't* go well," Hickson says, "and being committed to keeping these things from happening. This requires a willingness to understand that no single person runs the show."

5. **Help the patient provide informed consent.** Informed consent should be a discussion between the patient and the provider. The advocate facilitates that

discussion by ensuring that the patient receives sufficient information in understandable language and has an unpressured opportunity to ask questions and to have them answered.

Case Study 1-1:
Ospedale di Locarno, Switzerland, Improves Hand Hygiene Through a Pocket Bottle of Alcohol Solution

To reduce their rate of HAIs, Ospedale di Locarno's hygiene committee, in collaboration with the environment of care nosocomial infection prevention service, developed an educational program on hand hygiene that was implemented over a two-year period. In addition to providing some clear indications for alcohol-based hand disinfection (five indications for hand hygiene) and conducting clinical audits to determine the compliance among health care workers, Ospedale di Locarno introduced alcohol-based hand disinfection by making 100 ml bottles of alcohol-based solutions available to health care workers. Initial feedback from staff was positive, as having the bottle readily accessible made it easier and faster to perform hand hygiene. One initial shortcoming was the size of the bottle, because they took up a lot of space in the pockets of health care workers. When the campaign was launched, the vendor of the alcohol-based solution came up with the idea to provide a hook for hanging the bottle outside the pocket (*see* Case Study Figure 1). This innovation also made it easier and faster to dispense the product. The staff immediately showed their appreciation of the innovation, and today, nearly all health care workers are able to disinfect their hands anywhere in the hospital.

During implementation, Ospedale di Locarno observed that the consumption of 100 ml bottles had not increased on some wards, especially on the intensive care unit. During an inspection audit aimed at evaluating the issue, they found that the 100 ml bottle was considered to be superfluous on the wards where alcohol dispensers were available within close proximity (2 m) of the patient, as the health care worker did not need to walk a long way to perform hand hygiene. On the contrary, compliance was high on such patient care units as medicine and surgery, where beds are distributed over much longer distances. In these cases, the staff appreciated the innovation, as reported by the chief of nursing, "also because on these wards the alcohol hand-rub dispenser was located in the bathroom of the patient room, which is generally considered not to be a very clean place."

Case Study Figure 1-1.
Alcohol-based Solution Attached to Pocket

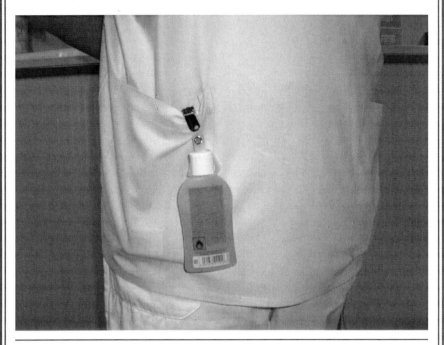

Alcohol-based solution attached to pocket.

Used with permission from Ospedale di Locarno, Switzerland.

During the first phase of introducing the hook for hanging bottles on the pockets of health care workers, Ospedale di Locarno distributed the bottles and hooks directly on the wards and during medical staff meetings. During the second phase, the bottles could be regularly ordered from pharmacy. "We have been handing out the bottle and hook during the staff induction program for some years now, and we explain to new staff the indications for hand hygiene and standard precautions," says the president of the hygiene committee. Moreover, everyone is invited to verify their hand-hygiene skills by using a special alcohol-based solution containing fluorescein, which becomes visible when exposed to a UV lamp. Health care workers thus have the possibility of immediately verifying their ability to appropriately perform alcohol-based hand hygiene.

More recently, another alcohol-based solution (an alcohol hand gel, which has a high content of protective substances) was introduced. Therefore, today staff can freely choose between the standard solution and the gel, based on their own preferences. "We believe it is important to let staff use the product they like the best," says the managing director. "We have also observed a reduction in the stains on the floors that were caused by alcohol drops falling to the floor."

By strongly promoting alcohol-based hand hygiene, Ospedale di Locarno recorded a small increase in staff with skin dryness issues who went to the occupational medicine service. In these instances, they advised staff to reduce hand washing with soap and water, which was believed to be the real cause of the problem. They also provided skin care and barrier creams when appropriate.

Evaluation

Following implementation, the pharmacy service observed a 15% increase in the consumption of the alcohol-based solution, while the nosocomial infection prevention service showed a 32% increase in compliance with hand hygiene and a greater than 90% compliance with the organization's policy of alcohol bottle proximity within 2 m.

With an eye toward continuing with staff education, every year, Ospedale di Locarno conducts randomized observational monitoring to measure compliance with hand hygiene and to provide immediate performance feedback to health care workers. Observational monitoring lasts at least 20 minutes and enables the organization to collect a number of data, including the adoption of standard precautions. "In this manner, we are able to come into direct contact with care providers and to educate them about good practices of infection control," says the infection control nurse. "However, in order to establish a good observational and educational climate, which has to be far from inspective, it is necessary to well inform the staff about what is going to be observed, what kind of feedback they will receive, and that their performance will not be disclosed to anybody else." On the contrary, all results are anonymous and are part of the data that are regularly published with the help of the quality department.

References

1. The Joint Commission: *High-Alert Medications: Strategies for Improving Safety.* Oakbrook Terrace, IL: Joint Commission Resources, 2008.
2. Institute for Healthcare Improvement: *What Should I Do if I See an Unsafe Condition or Behavior?* http://www.ihi.org/IHI/Programs/IHIOpenSchool/UnsafeConditionorBehavior.htm (accessed Jun. 12, 2009).
3. The Joint Commission: *Comprehensive Accreditation Manual for Hospitals: The Official Handbook.* Oakbrook Terrace, IL: Joint Commission Resources, 2009.
4. Joint Commission on Accreditation of Healthcare Organizations: *Patients as Partners: How to Involve Patients and Families in Their Own Care.* Oakbrook Terrace, IL: Joint Commission Resources, 2006.
5. Partnership for Clear Health Communication: Ask Me 3. http://www.npsf.org/askme3/ (accessed Dec. 29, 2008).
6. Joint Commission Resources: Strategies for improving health literacy. *Joint Commission Perspectives on Patient Safety* 8:8–9, Mar. 2008.
7. The Joint Commission: *"What Did the Doctor Say?:" Improving Health Literacy to Protect Patient Safety.* http://www.jointcommission.org/NR/rdonlyres/D5248B2E-E7E6-4121-8874-99C7B4888301/0/improving_health_literacy.pdf (accessed Jan. 30, 2009).
8. Villaire M., Mayer G.: *Dealing with Low-Literacy Patients.* Jan. 2008. http://www.physiciansnews.com/business/108villaire.html (accessed Jun. 12, 2009).
9. Dulak S.B.: A practical guide to a thorough history. RN Suppl:14–99; quiz 20–21, Jan. 2004.
10. Joint Commission Resources: How to be a patient advocate: Providing another layer of safety for patients. *Joint Commission Perspectives on Patient Safety* 7:11, Mar. 2007.

Chapter 2

Educating Nursing Staff on Safe Infection Prevention and Control Practices

Staff education in health care is changing. It is no longer a slide show with new rules and regulations twice a year in the staff break room; it is dynamic, it is every day, it is electronic, it is interactive, and it is immediate. The effective organization will embrace the challenge to get the necessary information to its nursing staff in the quest for improved patient safety and overall organizational performance.[1]

Prevention of health care–associated infections (HAIs) represents one of the major safety initiatives an organization can undertake, making the effective evaluation and possible redesign of existing infection prevention and control programs a priority.

The Joint Commission requires that organizations establish and implement goals for preventing HAIs within the organization based on prioritized risks and associated surveillance data. Interventions should include the following:
- Screening for exposure and/or immunity to infectious diseases that licensed independent practitioners, staff, student/trainees, and volunteers may come in contact with in their work environments
- Referral for assessment, potential testing, immunization and/or prophylaxis/treatment, and counseling as appropriate of licensed independent practitioners, staff, students/trainees, and volunteers who are identified as potentially having an infectious disease or risk of infectious disease that may put patients and other health care workers at risk
- Monitoring hand hygiene

Historically, health care systems have relied on infection prevention and control policies that recommend good hygiene through standard precautions[2] (*see* Table 2-1, page 24, for recommendations for applications of standard precautions). However, for these strategies to be effective, nurses and other health care workers must be

Table 2-1. Recommendations for Application of Standard Precautions in All Health Care Settings

Component	Recommendations
Hand hygiene	After touching blood, body fluids, secretions, excretions, contaminated items; immediately after removing gloves; between patient contacts; after using the restroom; and before eating
Gloves	For touching blood, body fluids, secretions, excretions, contaminated items; for touching mucous membranes and nonintact skin
Mask, eye protection (goggles), face shield*	During procedures and patient-care activities likely to generate splashes or sprays of blood, body fluids, secretions, especially suctioning, endotracheal intubation
Soiled patient-care equipment	Handle in a manner that prevents transfer of micro-organisms to others and to the environment; wear gloves if visibly contaminated; perform hand hygiene
Textiles and laundry	Handle in a manner that prevents transfer of micro-organisms to others and to the environment
Needles and other sharps	Do not recap, bend, break, or hand-manipulate used needles; if recapping is required, use a one-handed scoop technique only; use safety features when available; place used sharps in puncture-resistant container
Patient resuscitation	Use mouthpiece, resuscitation bag, other ventilation devices to prevent contact with mouth and oral secretions

* During aerosol-generating procedures on patients with suspected or proven infections transmitted by respiratory aerosols (e.g., SARS), wear a fit-tested N95 or higher respirator in addition to gloves, gown, and face/eye protection.

(continued)

Table 2-1. Recommendations for Application of Standard Precautions in All Health Care Settings, *continued*

Component	Recommendations
Patient placement	Prioritize for single-patient room if patient is at increased risk of transmission, is likely to contaminate the environment, does not maintain appropriate hygiene, or is at increased risk of acquiring infection or developing adverse outcome following infection
Respiratory hygiene/cough etiquette (source containment of infectious respiratory secretions in symptomatic patients, beginning at initial point of encounter [for example, triage and reception areas in emergency departments and physician offices])	Instruct persons to cover mouth/nose when sneezing/coughing; use tissues and dispose in no-touch receptacle; observe hand hygiene after soiling of hands with respiratory secretions; wear surgical mask if tolerated or maintain spatial separation, >3 feet if possible.

Source: Centers for Disease Control and Prevention: *Guidelines for Isolation Precautions: Presenting Transmission of Infectious Agents in Healthcare Settings 2007.* http://www.cdc.gov/ncidod/dhqp/pdf/guidelines/Isolation2007.pdf (accessed Feb. 23, 2009).

appropriately educated as to their application. In addition, protocols should be in place outlining the steps that nurses should take if they come in contact with an infectious patient or a potentially infectious patient.[2]

This chapter provides information on educating nurses about infection prevention and control practices. It includes initiatives developed by other organizations that relate to specific infection prevention and control topics.

Hand Hygiene

Hand hygiene is one of the most important measures health care workers can do to reduce the transmission of infection. Therefore, staff education about hand-hygiene protocols and procedures should be an integral part of any organization's infection prevention and control program.

Many HAIs are caused by pathogens transmitted between patients by nurses and other health care workers who have failed to clean their hands effectively.[3] Although it is widely known that patient-to-patient contact by way of unwashed hands is the principal route of transmission for most exogenously acquired infections, hand-hygiene compliance remains relatively low.[4] According to the Centers for Disease Control and Prevention (CDC), reasons for noncompliance may include the following[5]:

• Skin irritation caused by hand-hygiene agents
• Inaccessible hand-hygiene supplies
• Interference with health care worker–patient relationships
• Priority of care (that is, the patients' needs are given priority over hand hygiene)
• Wearing of gloves
• Forgetfulness
• Lack of knowledge of the guidelines
• Insufficient time for hand hygiene
• High workload and understaffing
• Lack of scientific information indicating a definitive impact of improved hand hygiene on HAI rates
• Lack of accountability

The Joint Commission gives organizations the option of complying with current World Health Organization (WHO) Hand-Hygiene Guidelines or CDC Hand-Hygiene Guidelines. To help organizations compare the two sets of guidelines, Joint Commission Resources has produced a crosswalk, which is a side-by-side comparison of the guidelines (*see* Figure 2-1, page 27).

To assist organizations with tracking hand-hygiene compliance with either the CDC or WHO guidelines, The Joint Commission has developed a hand-hygiene checklist, which is shown in Figure 2-2, page 30.

Tools for Educating Nursing Staff
A number of tools are available to help organizations educate nursing staff about good hand-hygiene practices, including the following:

• **Hand-hygiene course.** Developed by the CDC. Available at http://www.cdc.gov/handhygiene/training/interactiveEducation/.

Figure 2-1. CDC/WHO Hand-Hygiene Guidelines Crosswalk

World Health Organization (WHO) Hand Hygiene Guideline Recommendations
Comparison with Centers for Disease Control and Prevention (CDC) Guidelines

© 2007 Joint Commission Resources

I. Indications for handwashing and hand antisepsis

Recommendation	CDC Guideline	WHO Guideline	Key Points of WHO Guideline
A. Visible dirt, blood, or body fluids on hands of health care worker (HCW)	A. (IA) Non-antimicrobial or antimicrobial soap and water	A. (IB) Soap and water	Simplifies terminology and does not differentiate between non-antimicrobial and antimicrobial soap, unless specified
B. No visible dirt, blood, or body fluids on hands of HCW in the following clinical situations:	B. (IA) Prefer alcohol hand rub or alternatively, (IB) antimicrobial soap and water	B. (IA) Prefer alcohol hand rub or alternatively, (IB) soap and water	
1. Before direct patient contact	1. (IB) Recommend	1. (IB) Recommend before and after contact	Clarifies expanded use of hand hygiene
2. After removing gloves	2. (IB) Recommend	2. (IB) Recommend	
3. Before handling invasive device for insertion	3. (IB) Before donning sterile gloves for central venous catheter insertion; also for insertion of other invasive devices that do not require a surgical procedure using sterile gloves	3. (IB) Before insertion of all invasive devices, regardless of glove use	Clarifies clinical situations and simplifies terminology
4. After contact with blood, body fluids, mucous membranes, non-intact skin, and wound dressings	4. (IA) Recommend	4. (IA) Recommend	
5. Moving from contaminated patient body site to clean site during patient care	5. (II) Recommend	5. (IB) Recommend	
6. After contact with inanimate objects or medical equipment close to patient	6. (II) Recommend	6. (IB) Recommend	
C. Potential exposure to spore-forming organisms	C. (II) Non-antimicrobial or antimicrobial soap and water	C. (IB) Soap and water	Alcohol hand rub is ineffective against spore-forming organisms (for example, *Clostridium difficile, Bacillus anthracis*).
D. After using restroom	D. (IB) Non-antimicrobial or antimicrobial soap and water	D. (II) Soap and water	
E. Before handling medication or food	E. (IB) Non-antimicrobial or antimicrobial soap and water (before handling food)	E. (IB) Alcohol rub or soap and water (before handling both medication and food)	Recommends alcohol rub and expands recommendation to include medication
F. Concomitant or sequential use of alcohol rub with soap and water	F. No comment in non-surgical setting. In surgical (operating room) setting, recommend pre-washing hands with soap and water before alcohol rub (see III.G.2)	F. (II) Not recommended in either non-surgical or surgical setting	Pre-washing hands is not recommended.

II. Hand hygiene technique (non-surgical)

Recommendation	CDC Guideline	WHO Guideline	Key Points of WHO Guideline
A. Alcohol hand hygiene rub	A. (IB) Apply palmful, rub thoroughly until dry. Follow manufacturer's recommendation regarding volume of product to use	A. (IB) Apply palmful, rub thoroughly until dry. See instructional diagram.	Emphasizes hand hygiene technique rather than product volume and refers to diagram
B. Handwashing with soap and water. Wet hands first, wash thoroughly, rinse, dry with disposable towel, and use towel to turn off faucet	B. (IB) Wash for 15 seconds	B. (IB) Wash using vigorous rotational handrubbing technique. No time requirement. See instructional diagram.	Emphasizes hand hygiene technique rather than time requirement and refers to diagram
C. Avoid use of very hot water to decrease risk of dermatitis	C. (IB) Recommend	C. (IB) Recommend	
D. Dry hands thoroughly after hand hygiene	D. Recommend (see II.A and II.B)	D. Recommend; separate emphasis	
E. Avoid using multi-use (cloth) hand towels	E. (II) Recommend	E. (IB) Recommend	Emphasizes CDC recommendation regarding non-reuse of cloth towels by individuals

(continued)

Figure 2-1. CDC/WHO Hand-Hygiene Guidelines Crosswalk, *continued*

II. Hand hygiene technique (non-surgical) *(continued)*

Recommendation	CDC Guideline	WHO Guideline	Key Points of WHO Guideline
F. Use of antimicrobial-impregnated wipes as hand hygiene alternative	F. (IB) May use as alternative to non-antimicrobial soap and water. Do not use as alternative to antimicrobial soap and water or to alcohol hand rub	F. No comment	
G. Use of bar, liquid, leaf, or powder soaps. May use if using non-antimicrobial soap and water. Bar soap should be small size and sit on drainage rack.	G. (II) Recommend	G. (II) Recommend	

III. Surgical hand preparation

Recommendation	CDC Guideline	WHO Guideline	Key Points of WHO Guideline
A. Remove visible dirt before preparation	A. No comment	A: (II) Wash hands with soap and water	Emphasizes removal of visible dirt prior to surgical preparation
B. Clean fingernails using nail cleaner before preparation	B. (II) Recommend	B. (II) Recommend; clean under running water	
C. Design handwashing sink to minimize splashing	C. No comment	C. (II) Recommend	Recommends evaluating sink design; faulty faucet aerators have been associated with contamination of hand-washing water
D. Remove rings, watches, and bracelets before preparation	D. (II) Recommend	D. (II) Recommend	
E. Artificial nails prohibited	E. Recommend; for high-risk patients (e.g., in intensive-care unit or operating room)	E. (IA) Recommend; for direct contact with all patients	Expands prohibition of artificial nails; associated with changes in normal flora and impede proper hand hygiene
F. Type of surgical hand preparation: either antimicrobial soap and water or sustained activity alcohol rub	F. (IB) Recommend	F. (IB) Recommend; if water quality is not assured, use alcohol rub	Some areas may have water quality problems.
G. Duration and technique of surgical hand preparation			
1. If using antimicrobial soap and water	1. Manufacturer's recommendation; usually 2 to 6 minutes	1. Manufacturer's recommendation; usually 2 to 5 minutes	
2. If using alcohol rub	2. (IB) No time requirement. Pre-wash hands with antimicrobial soap and water.	2. (IB) No time requirement. Apply to dry hands and keep hands and forearms wet during application. Do not pre-wash hands or use alcohol rub and soap and water concomitantly or sequentially.	Pre-washing hands not recommended (see I.F)
H. Allow hands to dry thoroughly before gloving.	I. (IB) Recommend	I. (IB) Recommend	

IV. Selection of hand hygiene agents

Recommendation	CDC Guideline	WHO Guideline	Key Points of WHO Guideline
A. Administrative Actions			
1. Provide HCWs with efficacious (effective) product that is less likely to irritate.	1. (IB) Recommend	1. (IB) Recommend	
2. Maximize acceptance and solicit input from HCWs, and include cost as factor in product selection.	2. (IB) Recommend	2. (IB) Recommend	
3. Consult manufacturer's recommendation regarding possible interaction between a) product and gloves, and b) product and creams or lotions.	3. a. (II) Recommend b. (IB) Recommend	3. a. (II) Recommend b. (IB) Recommend	
B. Dispensers			
1. Access by HCWs: location of dispensers. For alcohol rub: recommend individual pocket-sized containers for HCWs	1. Refers to alcohol rub dispensers only; accessible at entrance to patient's room, at bedside, or other convenient locations.	1. (IB) Refers to both soap and alcohol rub dispensers; accessible at point of care.	Clarifies terminology and encourages flexibility in location
2. Function and deliver specified product volume	2. (II) Recommend	2. (II) Recommend	

(continued)

Figure 2-1. CDC/WHO Hand-Hygiene Guidelines Crosswalk, *continued*

IV. Selection of hand hygiene agents (continued)

Recommendation	CDC Guideline	WHO Guideline	Key Points of WHO Guideline
3. Alcohol rub product dispenser approved for flammable materials	3. (IC) Dispenser not specified but must store dispensers in cabinets approved for flammable materials.	3. (IC) Dispenser must be approved for flammable materials.	Clarifies flammability requirements for individual dispensers
4. Adding soap to partially filled dispensers for refill	4. (IA) Not recommended	4. (IA) Not recommended	Clean soap dispensers thoroughly before refilling to avoid bacterial contamination.
C. Skin Care			
1. Educate HCWs regarding hand hygiene practices that can reduce the risk of contact dermatitis, and provide creams and lotions	1. (IA) Recommend	(IA) Recommend	Provide alternatives for HCWs with allergic or adverse reactions to product

V. Use of gloves

Recommendation	CDC Guideline	WHO Guideline	Key Points of WHO Guideline
A. Gloves are not a substitute for hand hygiene	A. No comment	A. (IB) Recommend	Emphasizes use of hand hygiene after gloves are removed
B. Use gloves before contact with blood and body fluids, mucous membranes, and non-intact skin	B. (IC) Recommend	B. (IC) Recommend	
C. Remove gloves after contact with each patient and avoid re-use of gloves	C. (IB) Do not re-use the same gloves (or wash them between uses) with multiple patients.	C. (IB) If re-use is necessary, re-process gloves adequately between patients.	Glove reuse may be necessary in some areas. Recommends implementing a glove reprocessing method to maintain glove integrity while adequately cleaning gloves
D. Change or remove gloves if moving from contaminated to clean patient site or the environment	D. (II) Recommend	D. (II) Recommend	

VI. Other aspects of hand hygiene (non-surgical)

Recommendation	CDC Guideline	WHO Guideline	Key Points of WHO Guideline
A. Use of artificial nails/extenders	A. (IA) Prohibited for high-risk patients, e.g., in intensive care unit or operating room	A. (IA) Prohibited for all direct patient contact in all settings	Prohibition of artificial nails expanded (see III.E)
B. Nail length (natural nails); tips must be less than ¼ inch or 0.5 cm in length	B. (II) Recommend	B. (II) Recommend	
C. Wearing of rings in non-surgical health care settings	C. Unresolved issue	C. No comment	

Outcome Measures and Performance Indicators

Recommendation	CDC Guideline	WHO Guideline	Key Points of WHO Guideline
A. Monitoring of hand hygiene compliance			
1. Direct observation with HCW performance feedback; calculate number of hand hygiene episodes performed per number of opportunities.	1. Recommend	1. Recommend	
2. Indirect monitoring			
a. Monitor volume of product used for hand hygiene.	a. Calculate volume used per 1,000 patient-days.	a. Estimate volume used based on nursing activities	Estimate volume instead of calculating it.
b. Other monitoring	b. No comment	b. Count used paper towels.	Alternative monitoring
c. Electronic monitoring	c. No comment	c. Monitor use of sinks, hand hygiene product, or paper towels electronically.	Alternative monitoring
d. Monitor compliance with facility policies regarding jewelry, nail polish, and artificial nails.	d. Recommend non-specific monitoring	d. Monitor compliance by direct and indirect observation, self-assessment, and patient assessment	Specific measures to monitor compliance

For a downloadable version of this figure, please go to http://www.jcrinc.com/NRIC09/Extras/.

Figure 2-2. Hand-Hygiene Checklist for Joint Commission Compliance

Centers for Disease Control and Prevention Recommendations	World Health Organization Recommendations	Compliant Yes/No
I. Indications for Hand Washing and Hand Antisepsis		
A. Visible dirt, blood, or body fluids on hands of health care worker (HCW)	A. Soap and water	
B. No visible dirt, blood, or body fluids on hands of HCW in the following clinical situations: 1. Before direct patient contact 2. After removing gloves 3. Before handling invasive device for insertion 4. After contact with blood, body fluids, mucous membranes, non-intact skin, and wound dressings 5. Moving from contaminated patient body site to clean site during patient care 6. After contact with inanimate objects or medical equipment close to patient	B. Prefer alcohol hand rub or, alternatively, soap and water 1. Recommend before and after contact 2. Recommend 3. Before insertion of all invasive devices, regardless of glove use 4. Recommend 5. Recommend 6. Recommend	
C. Potential exposure to spore-forming organisms	C. Soap and water	
D. After using restroom	D. Soap and water	
E. Before handling medication or food	E. Alcohol rub or soap and water (before handling both medication and food)	
F. Concomitant or sequential use of alcohol rub with soap and water	F. Not recommended in either nonsurgical or surgical setting	
II. Hand Hygiene Technique (nonsurgical)		
A. Alcohol hand hygiene rub	A. Apply palmful, rub thoroughly until dry.	
B. Hand washing with soap and water. Wet hands first, wash thoroughly, rinse, dry with disposable towel, and use towel to turn off faucet.	B. Wash using vigorous rotational hand-rubbing technique. No time requirement.	
C. Avoid use of very hot water to decrease risk of dermatitis.	C. Recommend	
D. Dry hands thoroughly after hand hygiene.	D. Recommend; separate emphasis	
E. Avoid using multiuse (cloth) hand towels.	E. Recommend	
F. Use of antimicrobial-impregnated wipes as hand hygiene alternative	F. No comment	
G. Use of bar, liquid, leaf, or powder soaps. May use if using non-antimicrobial soap and water. Bar soap should be small size and sit on drainage rack.	G. Recommend	
III. Surgical Hand Preparation		
A. Remove visible dirt before preparation.	A. Wash hands with soap and water.	
B. Clean fingernails using nail cleaner before preparation.	B. Recommend; clean under running water.	
C. Design handwashing sink to minimize splashing.	C. Recommend	
D. Remove rings, watches, and bracelets before preparation.	D. Recommend	
E. Artificial nails prohibited	E. Recommend; for direct contact with all patients	
F. Type of surgical hand preparation: either antimicrobial soap and water or sustained activity alcohol rub	F. Recommend; if water quality is not assured, use alcohol rub.	
G. Duration and technique of surgical hand preparation: 1. If using antimicrobial soap and water 2. If using alcohol rub	G. 1. Manufacturer's recommendation; usually 2 to 5 minutes 2. No time requirement. Apply to dry hands and keep hands and forearms wet during application. Do not pre-wash hands or use alcohol rub and soap and water concomitantly or sequentially.	
H. Allow hands to dry thoroughly before gloving.	H. Recommend	

(continued)

Figure 2-2. Hand-Hygiene Checklist for
Joint Commission Compliance, *continued*

Centers for Disease Control and Prevention Recommendations	World Health Organization Recommendations	Compliant Yes/No
IV. Selection of Hand Hygiene Agents		

A. Administrative Actions
  1. Provide HCWs with efficacious (effective) product that is less likely to irritate.
  2. Maximize acceptance and solicit input from HCWs and include cost as factor in product selection.
  3. Consult manufacturer's recommendation regarding possible interaction between (a) product and gloves, and (b) product and creams or lotions.
	1. Recommend
	2. Recommend
	3a. Recommend
	3b. Recommend	

B. Dispensers
  1. Access by HCWs: location of dispensers. For alcohol rub: recommend individual pocket-sized containers for HCWs.
  2. Function and deliver specified product volume
  3. Alcohol rub product dispenser approved for flammable materials
  4. Adding soap to partially filled dispensers for refill
	1. Refers to both soap and alcohol rub dispensers; accessible at point of care.
	2. Recommend
	3. Dispenser must be approved for flammable materials.
	4. Not recommended	

C. Skin Care 1. Educate HCWs regarding hand hygiene practices that can reduce the risk of contact dermatitis and provide creams and lotions.	1. Recommend	
V. Use of Gloves		
A. Gloves are not a substitute for hand hygiene.	A. Recommend	
B. Use gloves before contact with blood and body fluids, mucous membranes, and non-intact skin.	B. Recommend	
C. Remove gloves after contact with each patient and avoid reuse of gloves.	C. If reuse is necessary, reprocess gloves adequately between patients.	
D. Change or remove gloves if moving from contaminated to clean patient site or the environment.	D. Recommend	
VI. Other Aspects of Hand Hygiene		
A. Use of artificial nails/extenders	A. Prohibited for all direct patient contact in all settings	
B. Nail length (natural nails); tips must be less than 1/4 inch or 0.5 cm in length.	B. Recommend	
C. Wearing of rings in nonsurgical health care settings	C. No comment	

The Joint Commission requires use of the CDC or WHO hand-hygiene guidelines. This checklist can help organizations to track compliance with hand-hygiene practices.

For a downloadable version of this figure, please go to http://www.jcrinc.com/NRIC09/Extras/.

- **CDC hand-hygiene poster** (*see* Figure 2-3, page 33).
- **Joint Commission Resources hand-hygiene posters.** Available for purchase at http://www.jcrinc.com/Other%2DResources/INFECTION%2DCONTROL%2 DHAND%2DHYGIENE%2DPOSTERS/248/.
- **PowerPoint slides with speaker notes.** Developed by the CDC. Available at http://www.cdc.gov/handhygiene/download/hand_hygiene_core.ppt#372,1,Slide 1.
- **"Hand Hygiene for Healthcare Workers" brochure.** Developed by Association for Professionals in Infection Control and Epidemiology (APIC). Available at http://www.apic.org/AM/Template.cfm?Section=Search&section=Brochures&tem plate=/CM/ContentDisplay.cfm&ContentFileID=8994.
- **"Glove Information for Healthcare Workers" brochure.** Developed by APIC. Available at http://www.apic.org/AM/Template.cfm?Section=Search&section= Brochures&template=/CM/ContentDisplay.cfm&ContentFileID=8989.

Surgical Site Infections

Surgical site infections (SSIs) are a common type of HAI, particularly in elderly or immunocompromised patients. Surgical procedures are becoming increasingly common, with nearly 30 million performed in the United States each year. As a result, SSIs are also on the rise, because any time a patient is "opened up," the risk exists for bacteria being introduced into the blood, tissues, and organs.[6] It is estimated that about 500,000 patients suffer from SSIs each year, which accounts for one quarter of all hospital-acquired infections.[7]

SSIs are particularly dangerous, because the patient's health may have already been compromised by the condition that required surgical treatment as well as the surgical procedure itself. Therefore, nurses need to take steps to ensure that the risk of an SSI is as low as possible—although this is a complex task.[6] "When you're trying to prevent infection, there are just so many things to control for," says Stephen Streed, M.S., C.I.C., system director, Epidemiology and Infection Control, Lee Memorial Health System, and a member of the Board of Directors of APIC.

This complexity is why one of the best defenses against SSIs is a structured infection prevention and control process that follows evidence-based practices—a process that all caregivers are aware of and can easily adhere to and that includes prevention measures to be taken before surgery, during the procedure, and postoperatively.[6] Following are some measures that such a process should include.

Figure 2-3. CDC Hand-Hygiene Poster

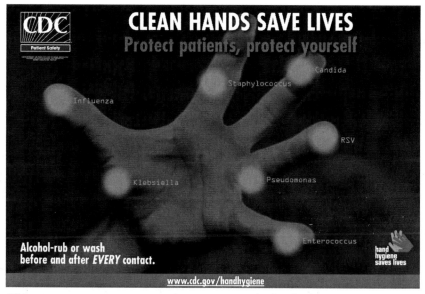

This poster can serve as a reminder to nurses and other health care workers about the importance of hand hygiene.

Source: Centers for Disease Control and Prevention. Available at http://www.cdc.gov/handhygiene/download/Hand_Hygiene_poster.pdf (accessed Dec. 2, 2009).

Before Surgery

Assess Other Infections. Patients about to have a surgical procedure should be checked for other types of infections—even those not at the operative site—such as urinary tract infections (UTIs) or skin infections. These infections have the potential to spread via the bloodstream and can attach to a foreign body implanted during surgery, such as an artificial joint or replaced valve, resulting in a serious infection that can be difficult to eradicate.[6] Nurses should be made aware of the signs and symptoms of infection and taught to assess patients for possible infections prior to surgery.

Use Clippers. In many cases, removing hair from the surgical site is not necessary. When hair removal is required, clippers should be used instead of razors. Razors should not be used, because they leave microscopic cuts on the skin that are all potential entry points for bacteria. This practice is such an important infection prevention and control issue that some hospitals have ensured the use of clippers by removing all razors from their operating rooms. Clippers should be used only by properly trained nurses or other staff members. Otherwise, they may still leave abrasions on the skin that could lead to infection.[6]

Administer Preventative Antimicrobial Agents. Many patients are given antimicrobial agents before surgery in an effort to prevent infections. Intravenous (IV) antimicrobial prophylaxis should be administered within 1 hour before incision (2 hours are allowed for the administration of vancomycin and fluoroquinolones). Prophylactic antimicrobial agents should be discontinued within 24 hours after surgery (within 48 hours is allowable for cardiothoracic procedures). The dose should also be adjusted for each patient, based on age, weight, and other criteria. For long procedures, patients may need to be redosed during surgery to maintain appropriate levels of antibiotics in the blood.[6] Because nurses are often responsible for administering these medications, they need to be educated about organizational protocols for antimicrobial prophylaxis administration.

To ensure that the preoperative antibiotic is given, some hospitals assign a certain surgical team member with the task; for example, the patient's preoperative nurse might be given the task of administering the antibiotic, so there is no question about whose responsibility it is, and it is easy to determine whether it was done.[8]

Prepare Skin. The goal of skin preparation is to remove as much potentially harmful bacteria as possible before the patient goes to surgery. Many hospitals have begun to use chlorhexidine (which has been used as a hand-hygiene product for many years) for this purpose, because it has a cumulative effect. "When you use chlorhexidine, you not only clean many of the microbes off the skin, but you prevent them from accumulating on the skin afterward," Streed explains. "Then when you use the product again, you remove even more of the harmful bacteria and reduce the amount that have the potential to get into the incision." Therefore, the patient may bathe with chlorhexidine the night before surgery and the day of the procedure.[6]

Nurses will need to be educated about how chlorhexidine should be used to pass this information along to their patients. Education should include the following instructions[9]:
• Before applying chlorhexidine, take a shower or bath using regular soap and water; rinse thoroughly.

- Apply the chlorhexidine to the entire body except for the face.
- Wash gently, but thoroughly, for five minutes, paying special attention to the surgical site; turn off the water while washing.
- Do not use regular soap after washing with chlorhexidine.
- Turn the water back on, and rinse thoroughly.
- Pat dry with a clean, dry towel.
- Do not apply lotion, powder, perfume, or aftershave after bathing.

During Surgery

Control Traffic. Nurses and other members of the surgical team should try to limit the number of people moving in and out of the operating room or procedure area during a surgical procedure. Each person who enters brings an additional risk of contamination. In addition, the opening and closing of doors causes air currents to swirl and to potentially sweep in bacteria from outside the operating room.[6]

Using Steam Sterilization. Most surgical instruments are sterilized using a long, thorough process that eradicates bacteria using steam or gas. However, on occasion, a particular instrument might be needed for a procedure shortly after it was used on a patient, so a shorter sterilization process using steam called flash sterilization is used.[6] According to The Joint Commission, the three critical steps of effectively sterilizing and reprocessing instruments include the following[10]:

1. **Cleaning and decontamination.** All visible soil must be removed prior to sterilization because steam and other sterilants cannot penetrate soil, particularly organic matter. Manufacturers' instructions are available for all instruments; these include directions for the cleaning and decontamination process. Some smooth metal instruments may be easily brushed clean, while complex products may require disassembly and special cleaning techniques. Many manufacturers specify that an enzymatic soak be used as well.

2. **Sterilization.** Most sterilization is accomplished via steam, but other methods are also available. Steam sterilization of all types, including flashing, must meet parameters (time, temperature and pressure) specified by both the manufacturer of the sterilizer, the maker of any wrapping or packaging, and the manufacturer of the surgical instrument. In addition to these instructions, parametric, chemical, and biological controls must be used as designed and directed by their manufacturers.

3. **Storage or return to the sterile field.** Each newly sterilized instrument must be carefully protected to ensure that it is not re-contaminated. For full steam sterilization cycles, packs of instruments are wrapped and sealed. Instruments

subjected to steam sterilization using methods other than full-cycle sterilization may be transported in "flash pans" or other devices specifically designed for the prevention of contamination during and after the steam process.

After Surgery

Maintain Sterile Dressing. The surgical incision should be covered with sterile dressing for at least 24 hours following surgery.

Be Aware of Patients with Risk Factors. Nurses should pay particular attention to high-risk patients. Patients with infection risk factors, such as diabetes, excess weight, smoking, or advanced age, should be assessed even more closely following a surgical procedure. Also, patients for whom all proper infection prevention and control measures could not be taken in unusual circumstances (such as an accident victim requiring emergency surgery) should be closely monitored for signs of infection. Because hyperglycemia increases risk for SSIs, particularly for major cardiac surgery and sternal wounds, blood-sugar levels should be watched and maintained in cardiac and intensive care unit (ICU) patients.[7,11]

Blood-glucose levels should be kept below 200 mg/dl for the first two days after surgery.[12] Nurses should be educated to measure blood-glucose level at 6:00 A.M. on postoperative day 1 and postoperative day 2, with the procedure day being postoperative day 0.[13]

Throughout the Hospital

To ensure that infection prevention and control procedures are implemented consistently and completely, organizations need to create processes that help prevent errors and omissions. For example, clearly assigning accountability for each step and requiring sign-offs can help caregivers maintain awareness of the process. Checklists can also help ensure that each measure is implemented as required, as can preassembled "kits" that include only the supplies and medications approved for infection prevention and control efforts.[6] "It's rare that a surgical-site infection occurs due to blatant negligence," says Susan Slavish, M.P.H., C.I.C., infection preventionist, Queen's Medical Center, and an infection prevention and control consultant for Joint Commission Resources. "If an error occurred, it's more likely that one of the infection control steps was just overlooked. This is why it's important to systemize and standardize these measures. When they become part of the overall procedure, and all caregivers are properly trained, it's much easier to ensure that all appropriate infection control measures have been taken and that the patient is as protected as possible."

Tools for Educating Nursing Staff About Surgical Site Infections

The following tools can help organizations educate nursing staff regarding how to reduce SSIs:

- **Getting Started Kit: Prevent Surgical Site Infections How-to Guide.** Developed by the Institute for Healthcare Improvement (IHI). Available at http://www.ihi.org/ nr/rdonlyres/c54b5133-f4bb-4360-a3e4-2952c08c9b59/0/ssihowtoguide.doc.
- **PowerPoint Presentation with Facilitator Notes.** Developed by the IHI. Available at http://www.ihi.org/NR/rdonlyres/0084A14D-03E2-4BA9-B226-792B35CD34D1/ 0/SSIPresentationwithFacilitatorNotesFeb2008.ppt.
- *Strategies to Prevent Surgical Site Infections in Acute Care Hospitals.* SHEA/IDSA practice recommendation. Available at http://www.journals.uchicago.edu/doi/pdf/ 10.1086/591064.

Multidrug-Resistant Organisms

Multidrug-resistant organisms (MDROs) are organisms that have developed resistance to most antibiotics, most often because of their overuse.[13] Examples include "spider bites" that refuse to heal, "shoulder sprains" that progress to respiratory failure, and skin infections that turn into deadly bone infections in just a few short days. In addition, the news has been flush with stories of "superbugs" that threaten life and limb.

According to the CDC, the proportion of bacteria that are resistant to antibiotics has increased dramatically in recent decades. A good example is *Staphylococcus aureus,* the bacteria that causes "staph" infections. Between 1972 and 2004, the proportion of drug-resistant staph bacteria increased from 2% to 63%. Now, methicillin-resistant *Staphylococcus aureus* (MRSA) is a leading concern for infection preventionists. Other drug-resistant organisms on the rise include vancomycin-resistant *enterococci* (VRE) and *Clostridium difficile (C. diff)*.[14–16]

All nursing staff should receive education about MDROs during orientation and regularly thereafter.[17] Education should include the following topics[17]:

- The epidemiology and risks of MDROs
- Identification, prevention, and control, with an emphasis on the nurse's role
- The organization's previous experience in managing MDROs
- Specific processes, such as contact or isolation precautions
- How to report problems or suggest improvements

Tools for Educating Nurses About MDROs

The following tools can help organizations educate nursing staff on how to prevent and control MDROs:

- **Complimentary MDRO Toolkit** available at http://www.jcrinc.com/MDRO-Toolkit/. Soule B., Weber S.: *What Every Health Care Executive Should Know: The Cost of Antibiotic Resistance.* Oakbrook Terrace, IL: Joint Commission Resources, 2009.
- The Joint Commission: *Staff Pocket Guide to MDROs.* Oakbrook Terrace, IL: Joint Commission Resources, 2009.

Methicillin-Resistant Staphylococcus Aureus *(MRSA)*

The rising incidence of HAIs caused by MRSA, the most prevalent antibiotic-resistant pathogen in many parts of the world, is of increasing concern. In 1980, MRSA accounted for only 2% of all *S. aureus* HAIs reported in National Nosocomial Infections Surveillance system (NNIS) hospitals.[2] MRSA currently accounts for 40% to 60% of *S. aureus* infections.[2]

As part of its "5 Million Lives" campaign, IHI recommends that organizations provide the following five key components of care[18]:

1. **Hand hygiene** (*see* Hand Hygiene on page 25).
2. **Decontamination of environment and equipment.** If not properly disinfected between patients, medical equipment can be a source of transmission of pathogens between patients.[20] Every item that comes into contact with the patient, from bedside commodes to blood-glucose meters and stethoscopes, should be cleaned between patients.[19] An important way to reduce the risk of environmental factors transmitting infection is to educate nurses about their parts in infection prevention and control.[19]
3. **Active surveillance.** As the incidence of MRSA has increased, so, too, have concerns about persons who unknowingly may be colonized with the organism. Colonization may have occurred at a hospital, another health care facility, or even an unknown location in the community. When colonized individuals are admitted to the hospital, they become another potential source for transmission. Some hospitals perform active surveillance cultures (ASCs) to identify colonized patients on admission. Hospitals typically begin this screening in high-risk populations, such as those in the ICU or those meeting high-risk criteria. Guidelines from the CDC Healthcare Infection Control Practices Advisory Committee (HICPAC) do not currently provide a definitive recommendation

and suggest only that ASCs be "considered . . . if other control measures have been ineffective," leaving that determination to the organization. Several states have legislation pending or approved that requires screening of patients.[18] Nurses should be aware of the organization's surveillance protocols, including steps to take if a patient is colonized or infected.

4. **Contact precautions.** As with hand hygiene, the recommendations for contact precautions are not new and have been in the CDC guidelines for years. Contact precautions should be implemented routinely for all patients colonized or infected with MRSA.[14] In long term care facilities, contact precautions can be modified to allow colonized/infected patients whose site of colonization or infection can be appropriately contained and who can observe good hand-hygiene practices to enter common areas and to participate in group activities.[13] Nurses should receive training in contact precautions, including education about the organization's protocol for when contact precautions should be initiated.

Conflicting evidence exists about when contact precautions should be discontinued for patients treated for MRSA. The CDC recommends that contact precautions be discontinued when three or more surveillance cultures are repeatedly negative over the course of one or two weeks, particularly if the patient does not have a draining wound or other condition that might allow for easy transmission to another patient.[13] Nurses should be made aware of the organization's policy for discontinuing contact precautions.

An important aspect of ensuring reliable compliance with contact precautions is ensuring that supplies are always readily available and accessible. Gowns and gloves (in multiple sizes) should be at the point of care, in stock, and placed in consistent and visible locations. Nurses or other health care workers who must go looking for supplies are less likely to use them routinely.[18]

Private rooms are recommended as the ideal in most guidelines, with acknowledgment that this is not always possible. Cohorting of patients is the next recommended approach when private rooms are not available. Because rooms may not be available, and moving patients poses its own set of challenges and opportunities for error, organizations are identifying other ways to ensure that contact precautions are used appropriately. For example, some hospitals are marking a "zone" around the patient bed (a painted line or tape on the floor) indicating an area in which contact precautions must be used. If anyone crosses the line, he or she must don gown and gloves.[18]

5. **Device bundles.** Invasive devices are well known to be potential sources for infection, as they bypass natural defenses; this is particularly true in critical care settings, where patients are further compromised by their illnesses or injuries. Patients with central lines or who are receiving mechanical ventilation may develop device-related infections from MRSA if they are already colonized with the organism or if it is transmitted to them during their hospitalization. Minimizing device days is essential to reducing the risk of device-related infection. Another strategy is the use of "bundles" for patients who have central lines or who are on ventilators—that is, groupings of best practices that individually improve care but when applied together result in substantially greater improvement. Many hospitals that have used central-line and ventilator bundles (*see* Central Line–Associated Bloodstream Infections on page 47 and Ventilator-Associated Pneumonia on page 56) have seen significant reductions in central line–associated bloodstream infections (CLABSIs) and ventilator-associated pneumonia (VAP) from all organisms. Implementing these device bundles is another effective strategy for nursing staff to decrease HAIs from MRSA and other organisms.[18]

Tools for Educating Nurses About MRSA
The following tools can help educate nursing staff about MRSA:
- *PowerPoint Presentation: Reduce Methicillin-Resistant* Staphylococcus aureus *(MRSA) Infection.* Developed by the IHI. Available at http://www.ihi.org/NR/rdonlyres/B4CB8709-BD6B-479E-9E9E-A7D04A51BF4E/0/MRSAIntroSlidesFeb2008.ppt#508,1,Reduce Methicillin-Resistant Staphylococcus aureus (MRSA) Infection.
- **Getting Started Kit: Reduce Methicillin-Resistant *Staphylococcus aureus* (MRSA) Infection How-to Guide.** Developed by the IHI. Available at http://www.ihi.org/nr/rdonlyres/f4d9de7a-3952-4ae7-bbac-4e4222084a03/0/mrsahowtoguide.doc.
- **"Don't Open the Door to Infection" Poster** (*see* Figure 2-4, page 41).

Vancomycin-Resistant Enterococci
Reports of VRE have increasingly appeared over the past few years.[20] Outbreaks of VRE colonization or infection have usually involved high-risk patient populations,

Figure 2-4. Don't Open the Door to Infection

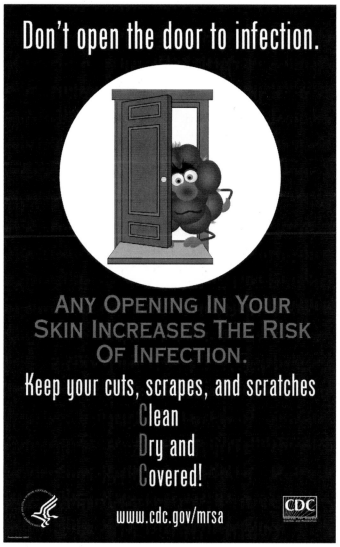

This poster can help remind staff to keep cuts clean, dry, and covered.

Source: Centers for Disease Control and Prevention. Available at http://www.cdc.gov/ncidod/dhqp/pdf/ar/mrsaPosters/DontOpenDoor.pdf (accessed Dec. 2, 2009).

such as those in ICUs and kidney, oncology, and transplant patients. The most important reservoirs for VRE are the gastrointestinal tracts of patients and contaminated environmental surfaces.

Enterococci, while not usually virulent in patients at normal risk, can remain dormant and unnoticed for long periods within patients (high ratio of colonization to infection) and on environmental surfaces.[20] According to the CDC, VRE may be spread by health care workers through inadequate hand hygiene or through contact with items, such as bedrails, sinks, faucets, and doorknobs.[21]

Educating Nursing Staff About VRE

Recently reported successes in controlling VRE outbreaks share five action recommendations. Staff and licensed independent practitioner education should include the following instructions[13,20,21]:

1. **Limit vancomycin use.** Although most nurses do not prescribe medications, they can help educate patients about the appropriate use of antibiotics. Nurses should be educated about the proper use of vancomycin (*see* Sidebar 2-1, page 43) so they might effectively intervene for their patients if necessary.
2. **Set up rigorous surveillance-culturing systems.** Keep careful records of all demographic data, hospital history, and outcomes. Each organization should determine who and when to screen for VRE.
3. **Give in-service training to housekeeping personnel, nurses, and physicians.** Support education by posting CDC guidelines on appropriate use of vancomycin and protocols for isolation and cleaning.
4. **Clean all environmental surfaces through an aggressive environmental decontamination program.** Prioritize room cleaning for patients who are on contact precautions. The main focus should be on cleaning and disinfecting frequently touched surfaces (for example, bedrails, bedside commodes, bathroom fixtures in the patient's room, doorknobs) and equipment in the patient's immediate vicinity.
5. **Institute barrier isolation to prevent transmission of infections.** This process may involve isolation of individuals or cohorting of colonized patients.

Clostridium Difficile

Morbidity and mortality rates related to *Clostridium difficile*–associated disease (CDAD) are increasing. The NNIS system tracked a significant increase in CDAD rates from the late 1980s through 2001,[15] and the CDC found that the number

Sidebar 2-1.

CDC Guidelines on the Appropriate Use of Vancomycin

The following are situations in which the use of vancomycin is appropriate or acceptable:

- For treatment of serious infections caused by beta-lactam-resistant gram-positive micro-organisms. Vancomycin may be less rapidly bactericidal than beta-lactam agents for beta-lactam-susceptible staphylococci.
- For treatment of infections caused by gram-positive micro-organisms in patients who have serious allergies to beta-lactam antimicrobials.
- When antibiotic-associated colitis fails to respond to metronidazole therapy or is severe and potentially life threatening.
- Prophylaxis, as recommended by the American Heart Association, for endocarditis following certain procedures in patients at high risk for endocarditis.
- Prophylaxis for major surgical procedures involving implantation of prosthetic materials or devices (for example, cardiac and vascular procedures or total hip replacement) at institutions that have high rates of infections caused by MRSA or methicillin-resistant *Staphylococcus epidermidis.* A single dose of vancomycin administered immediately before surgery is sufficient unless the procedure lasts more than six hours, in which case the dose should be repeated. Prophylaxis should be discontinued after a maximum of two doses.

The following are situations in which the use of vancomycin should be discouraged:

- Routine surgical prophylaxis, other than in a patient who has a life-threatening allergy to beta-lactam antibiotics.
- Empiric antimicrobial therapy for a febrile neutropenic patient, unless initial evidence indicates that the patient has an infection caused by gram-positive micro-organisms (for example, at an inflamed exit site of catheter), and the prevalence of infections caused by MRSA in the hospital is substantial.

(continued)

Sidebar 2-1.

CDC Guidelines on the Appropriate Use of Vancomycin, *continued*

- Treatment in response to a single blood culture positive for coagulase-negative staphylococcus, if other blood cultures taken during the same time frame are negative (that is, if contamination of the blood culture is likely). Because contamination of blood cultures with skin flora (for example, *S. epidermidis*) could result in inappropriate administration of vancomycin, phlebotomists and other personnel who obtain blood cultures should be trained to minimize microbial contamination of specimens.
- Continued empiric use for presumed infections in patients whose cultures are negative for beta-lactam-resistant gram-positive micro-organisms.
- Systemic or local (for example, antibiotic lock) prophylaxis for infection or colonization of indwelling central or peripheral intravascular catheters.
- Selective decontamination of the digestive tract.
- Eradication of MRSA colonization.
- Primary treatment of antibiotic-associated colitis.
- Routine prophylaxis for very low-birth-weight infants (that is, infants who weigh less than 1,500 g [3 lbs. 4 oz.])
- Routine prophylaxis for patients on continuous ambulatory peritoneal dialysis or hemodialysis.
- Treatment (chosen for dosing convenience) of infections caused by beta-lactam-sensitive gram-positive micro-organisms in patients who have renal failure.
- Use of vancomycin solution for topical application or irrigation.

To enhance compliance with recommendations, key parameters of vancomycin use can be monitored through the hospital's quality assurance/improvement process or as part of the drug-utilization review of the pharmacy and therapeutics committee and the medical staff.

Source: Centers for Disease Control and Prevention.

and the rate of hospitalized patients discharged with CDAD increased from 2000 to 2003.[16]

The Joint Commission requires that organizations implement evidence-based practices to prevent HAIs due to MDROs. Careful use of antibiotics is an important step health care professionals can take to prevent the spread of CDAD. "The *C. difficile* problem has brought some of the problems with antibiotic prescribing closer to home," explains L. Clifford McDonald, M.D., a medical epidemiologist in the Division of Healthcare Quality Promotion, National Center for Infectious Diseases, at the CDC. "A lot of patients and clinicians see antibiotic resistance as a societal problem rather than one that could affect them. But with CDAD, it's a per-use risk: The patient who gets [a high-risk] antibiotic is going to be at increased risk for disease that can lead to multiple occurrences, prolonged hospital stays, higher costs, and possibly severe complications requiring colectomy or resulting in death." Although most nurses do not prescribe antibiotics, they can help teach patients why antibiotics will not cure viral infections and how taking antibiotics when they are not necessary can actually cause them harm.

C. diff can be spread from person to person or through contact with a contaminated surface. Thus, organizations caring for patients who have already been diagnosed with CDAD should establish procedures to inhibit outbreaks. Nurses should then be educated as to the appropriate procedures. The following measures can help organizations establish safety processes:

- Use contact precautions, including placing patients in private rooms or in rooms with other CDAD patients.
- Because alcohol-based hand rubs are not effective against *C. diff*, it is recommended that hands be washed before and after gloving, and personal protective equipment, such as gowns and goggles, should be used as needed when caring for patients with *C. diff*.
- It is advisable to use disposable equipment or dedicate reusable equipment for individual patients with CDAD. Because *C. diff* spores can survive up to five months within the environment of care, everything in that environment—including beds, telephones, toilets, medical equipment, and floors and work surfaces—should be cleaned and disinfected regularly with diluted bleach. (Quaternary ammonium and phenolic disinfectants are not able to inactivate *C. diff* spores.)

Catheter-Associated Urinary Tract Infections

UTIs are a common type of HAI, accounting for more than 40% of the total number reported by acute care hospitals and affecting an estimated 600,000 patients per year.[22] Between 66% and 86% of hospital-acquired UTIs are caused by instrumentation of the urinary tract, mainly urinary catheterization.[22] Though data is limited, UTIs are of particular concern in long term care, home care, and other care settings as well. Although not all catheter-associated urinary tract infections (CAUTIs) can be prevented, a large number could likely be avoided by proper management of indwelling catheters.

An estimated four million patients each year are subjected to urinary catheterization and, therefore, are at risk for CAUTIs.[22] One of the most important infection prevention and control measures is to limit the use of urinary catheters to carefully selected patients. Generally, urinary catheterization is indicated for the following reasons[22]:

- To relieve urinary tract obstruction
- To permit urinary drainage in patients with neurogenic bladder dysfunction and urinary retention
- To aid in urologic surgery or other surgery on contiguous structures
- To obtain accurate measurements of urinary output in critically ill patients

Nurses should learn that urinary catheterization should not be used to obtain urine for culture or for other diagnostic tests when the patient can voluntarily void. It should also not be used as a substitute for convenience in the incontinent patient.[22]

When educating nursing staff about the prevention of CAUTIs, the CDC recommends that the following elements be included in all programs[22]:

- Emphasize hand hygiene.
- Catheterize only when necessary.
- Insert the catheter using aseptic technique and sterile equipment.
- Secure the catheter properly.
- Maintain a closed sterile drainage.
- Obtain urine samples aseptically.
- Maintain unobstructed urine flow.
- Use the smallest suitable bore catheter.
- Avoid irrigation unless needed to prevent or to relieve obstruction.
- Do not change catheters at arbitrary fixed intervals.

Tools for Educating Nursing Staff About the Prevention of CAUTIs

The following tools can help educate nursing staff about how to prevent CAUTIs:

• **Catheter-Associated Urinary Tract Infections (CAUTI): Fact Sheet.** Developed by the Wound Ostomy and Continence Nurses Society. Available at http://www.wocn.org/pdfs/WOCN_Library/Fact_Sheets/cauti_fact_sheet.pdf.

• **"Preventing Catheter-Associated Urinary Tract Infections (CAUTIs)" Brochure.** Developed by Bard Medical Division. Available at http://www.bardmedical.com/resources/product/brochures/Complete%20Care%20White%20Paper%200509-12.pdf.

Central Line–Associated Bloodstream Infections

Approximately 48% of all ICU patients have central lines, which equates to about 15 million central-venous-catheter-days per year.[23] Around 5.3 CLABSIs occur per 1,000 catheter-days in ICUs.[23] The attributable mortality for such central-line infections is approximately 18%, which translates to around 14,000 deaths annually due to central-line infections.[23] Some estimates put this figure as high as 28,000 deaths per year.[23]

CLABSIs can largely be prevented through the use of a "bundle" of five care steps. These include the following[23,24]:

1. Use proper hand hygiene.
2. Use maximal barrier precautions for the clinician (sterile gown, mask, gloves, hair covering) and the patient (sterile drape).
3. Choose an optimal insertion site (the subclavian vein is the preferred site for nontunneled catheters).
4. Cleanse the insertion site with chlorhexidine skin antisepsis.
5. Monitor the site daily, and promptly remove unnecessary lines.

The Joint Commission requires that organizations implement best practices or evidence-based guidelines to prevent CLABSIs. Staff should be educated about the appropriate frequency of replacement for catheters, dressings, administration sets, and fluids to prevent CLABSIs. The CDC has developed guidelines (*see* Figure 2-5, page 48).

Figure 2-5. Summary of Recommended Frequency of Replacement for Catheters, Dressings, Administration Sets, and Fluids

Catheter	Replacement and relocation of device	Replacement of catheter site dressing	Replacement of administration sets	Hang time for parenteral fluids
Peripheral venous catheters	In *adults*, replace catheter and rotate site no more frequently than every 72–96 hours. Replace catheters inserted under emergency basis and insert a new catheter at a different site within 48 hours. In *pediatric* patients, do not replace peripheral catheters unless clinically indicated.	Replace dressing when the catheter is removed or replaced, or when the dressing becomes damp, loosened, or soiled. Replace dressings more frequently in diaphoretic patients. In patients who have large bulky dressings that prevent palpation or direct visualization of the catheter insertion site, remove the dressing and visually inspect the catheter at least daily and apply a new dressing.	Replace intravenous tubing, including add-on devices, no more frequently than at 72-hour intervals unless clinically indicated. Replace tubing used to administer blood, blood products, or lipid emulsions within 24 hours of initiating the infusion. *No recommendation* for replacement of tubing used for intermittent infusions. Consider short extension tubing connected to the catheter to be a portion of the device. Replace such extension tubing when the catheter is changed.	*No recommendation* for the hang time of intravenous fluids, including nonlipid-containing parenteral nutrition fluids. Complete infusion of lipid-containing parenteral nutrition fluids (e.g., 3-in-1 solutions) within 24 hours of hanging the fluid. Complete infusion of lipid emulsions alone within 12 hours of hanging the fluid. Complete infusions of blood products within 4 hours of hanging the product.
Midline catheters	*No recommendation* for the frequency of the catheter replacement.	As above.	As above.	As above.
Peripheral arterial catheters	In *adults*, do not replace catheters routinely to prevent catheter-related infection. In *pediatric* patients, *no recommendation* for the frequency of catheter replacement. Replace disposable or reusable transducers at 72-hour intervals. Replace continuous flush device at the time the transducer is replaced.	Replace dressing when the catheter is replaced, or when the dressing becomes damp, loosened, or soiled, or when inspection of the site is necessary.	Replace the intravenous tubing at the time the transducer is replaced (i.e., 72-hour intervals).	Replace the flush solution at the time the transducer is replaced (i.e., 72-hour intervals).

(continued)

This chart can be used to educate staff about how frequently catheters, dressings, administration sets, and fluids should be changed to prevent CLABSIs.

Figure 2-5. Summary of Recommended Frequency of Replacement for Catheters, Dressings, Administration Sets, and Fluids, *continued*

Catheter	Replacement and relocation of device	Replacement of catheter site dressing	Replacement of administration sets	Hang time for parenteral fluids
Central venous catheters including peripherally inserted central catheters and hemodialysis catheters	**Do not routinely replace catheters.**	Replace gauze dressings every 2 days and transparent dressings every 7 days on short-term catheters. Replace the dressing when the catheter is replaced, or when the dressing becomes damp, loosened, or soiled, or when inspection of the site is necessary.	Replace intravenous tubing and add-on devices no more frequently than at 72-hour intervals. Replace tubing used to administer blood products or lipid emulsions within 24 hours of initiating the infusion.	*No recommendation* for the hang time of intravenous fluids, including nonlipid-containing parenteral nutrition fluids. Complete infusions of lipid-containing fluids within 24 hours of hanging the fluid.
Pulmonary artery catheters	**Do not replace catheter to prevent catheter-related infection.**	As above.	As above.	As above.
Umbilical catheters	**Do not routinely replace catheters.**	Not applicable.	Replace intravenous tubing and add-on devices no more frequently than at 72-hour intervals. Replace tubing used to administer blood products or lipid emulsions within 24 hours of initiating the infusion.	*No recommendation* for the hang time of intravenous fluids, including nonlipid-containing parenteral nutrition fluids. Complete infusion of lipid-containing fluids within 24 hours of hanging the fluid. Includes nontunneled catheters, tunneled catheters, and totally implanted devices.

Source: Centers for Disease Control and Prevention.

Figure 2-6. Central Line Insertion Care Team Checklist

Central Line Insertion
Care Team Checklist
➤ If any item on the checklist is **not** adhered to or there are any concerns, contact the ICU attending

Purpose:	To work as a team to decrease patient harm from catheter-related blood stream infections
When:	During **all** central venous or **central** arterial line insertions or re-wires
By whom:	Bedside nurse

If there is an observed violation of infection control practices, line placement should stop immediately and the violation should be corrected. If a correction is required, mark yes to question #6 *and explain violation at the bottom of the page and what corrections were made*

Patient's name or Room Number_____

1. Today's date _____ / _____ / _____
2. Is the procedure: ☐ Elective ☐ Emergent
3. Procedure: ☐ New line ☐ Rewire
4. Site Rite Used: ☐ Yes ☐ No ☐ Internal Jugular ☐ Subclavian ☐ Femoral
   If equipment is available, ultrasound guidance should be used for all non-emergent internal jugular line placements. (Optional for subclavian and femoral line placement.)

	Yes	Yes After correction	Don't Know
5. **Before the procedure,** did the house staff:			
Perform a **"time-out"**	☐	☐	
Wash hands (chlorhexidine or soap) immediately prior	☐	☐	**(ask if needed)**
Was hand washing directly observed?	☐	☐	
Place pt in trendelenburg position (< 0 degrees)	☐	☐	to prevent air embolism
Sterilize procedure site (chorhexidine)	☐	☐	☐
Drape entire patient in a sterile fashion	☐	☐	☐
During the procedure, did the house staff:			
Use hat, mask, sterile gown and gloves	☐	☐	☐
Maintain a sterile field	☐	☐	☐
Did all personnel assisting follow the above precautions	☐	☐	☐
Ensure line aspirates blood to prevent hemothorax	☐	☐	
Transduce CVP or estimate CVP by fluid column	☐	☐	
After the procedure:			
Was a sterile dressing applied to the site	☐	☐	☐

	Yes	No
6. **Was a correction required to ensure compliance with Safety & Infection control practices? Explain.**		

Please return completed form to the designated location in your area

Version 12/2004

The use of a checklist, such as this one, can help organizations monitor staff compliance with policies to prevent CLABSIs.

Source: Central Line Insertion Care Team Checklist. http://www.ihi.org/NR/rdonlyres/65DFE617-F6A3-4851-82F7-BD02FEA9E86B/0/PronovostCentralLineBSIchecklist1204.doc. Used with permission by Peter Pronovost, M.D.

Tools for Educating Nursing Staff About the Prevention of CLABSIs

The following tools can help educate nursing staff about how to prevent CLABSIs:

- **Getting Started Kit: Prevent Central Line Infections How-to Guide.** Developed by the IHI. Available at http://www.ihi.org/nr/rdonlyres/0ad706aa-0e76-457b-a4b0-78c31a5172d8/0/centrallineinfectionshowtoguide.doc.
- **PowerPoint Presentation with Facilitator Notes.** Developed by the IHI. Available at http://www.ihi.org/NR/rdonlyres/225E0F9A-19AD-445E-A0B6-1D1413FD9780/0/CentralLinesPresentationwithFacilitatorNotesOct2008.ppt.
- **Central Line Insertion Care Team Checklist** (*see* Figure 2-6, page 50).

Case Study 2-1:
Sutter Roseville Medical Center

In January 2006, Sutter Roseville Medical Center (SRMC) set out to convert its current IV team to an advanced vascular access team. "We had a couple of issues that we were dealing with," says Sophie Harnage, R.N., B.S.N., clinical manager, Infusion Services, Sutter Roseville Medical Center, Roseville, California. "One was infections. The other was preservation of venous access."

Prior to development of the advanced vascular access team, peripheral access and centrally inserted central catheters (CICCs) were the primary route for IV administration at SRMC.[27] "We began by collecting data from a variety of sources and looking at evidence of best practices, including CDC and IHI recommendations," says Harnage. The IV team then reviewed its policies and procedures and correlated them with what it found in the literature. It also reviewed all the products it was currently using and new products that were on the market.

"Next, we wanted to make sure we were providing the most appropriate vascular access device for each patient within 24 to 48 hours of admission to meet the patient's needs," Harnage says. "This, in turn, would reduce VAD [vascular access device] complications, increase reliability and consistency, promote patient safety and comfort, and improve patient satisfaction. Placing the appropriate device the first time preserves the patient's vascular status."

The advanced vascular access team at SRMC next developed a bundle of procedures to be used for central-line insertion and maintenance. "Our purpose was to develop a clinical bundle that would reduce catheter-related bloodstream infections," says Harnage. "In order to accomplish this goal, we had to change practice throughout our facility related to the insertion and management of all central lines." SRMC's central-line bundle has seven components, which include the following[26]:

1. Maximum barrier precautions using a custom barrier kit for every central-line insertion.
2. Ultrasound-guided peripherally inserted central catheter (PICC) insertion. "The upper arm basilic vein is the vein of choice," Harnage says.
3. The use of antimicrobial interventions (for example, cleansing the site with alcohol and disinfecting with chlorhexidine gluconate (CHG) prior to insertion, and placing a protective disk with CHG directly on the insertion site after insertion).
4. The use of a neutral connector device, which reduces reflux and supports SRMC's saline-only flushing protocol.
5. Septum disinfection.
6. A protocol for catheter flushing.
7. Daily monitoring of all central lines by the vascular access team.

Staff Education

Newly hired team members are given a six-week orientation. Orientation consists of the following:

- One-on-one training with an experienced PICC R.N., including demonstrated competency of PICC placement.
- Review of SRMC's vascular access policies and procedures.
- Training on early assessment for appropriate VAD with review of Infusion Nurse's Society and CDC standards.
- A class on radiologic interpretation of chest films for PICC tip verification. "Everyone who takes the course must demonstrate competency by passing a written test and successfully reading 10 chest films for tip placement," Harnage says.

The team continues to provide ongoing education to the house staff on a daily basis. "We're not just a PICC, stick, and run team," Harnage says. "We conduct monthly staff meetings and revise policies and procedures. We have a whole educational piece, too." Ongoing education efforts include the following:

- A colorful grid to remind staff of proper flushing protocols.
- Educational cards placed on all medication carts as bundle-compliance reminders or review for house staff. "One particular card describes step-by-step the procedure on changing a central-line dressing," Harnage says (*see* Figure 2-7, page 54).
- Hospitalwide in-service courses on central-line care and maintenance. "These in-services, in addition to hospitalwide audits, help ensure compliance with our catheter care and flushing protocols," says Harnage.
- Posters with helpful hints and reminders for nurses to flush their lines or swab their hubs before accessing.
- Daily monitoring of all central lines so that if issues arise, the team can intervene early to support one another and to correct the problems.

Harnage admits that some were initially resistant to change. "Whenever you initiate a new product or practice, there is always some resistance," she says. "As our team was growing and expanding, we overcame this challenge through diligent staff support and education. Physician acceptance was driven by reduced infection rates and significant workload alleviation. For example, the PICC team now places most of the central lines at SRMC, a responsibility that was previously solely on the physicians."

Evaluation

The vascular access team is required to complete a central-line-insertion-procedure (CLIP) form (*see* Figure 2-8, page 55) for each central-line insertion. The completed forms are sent to infection prevention and control and are used as audit tools to ensure bundle compliance and to determine whether additional staff education is needed.

The advanced vascular access team has inserted more than 6,000 PICC lines, using the central-line bundle for every insertion since its implementation in 2006, and has had zero CLABSIs. "Our central-line bundle demonstrated the benefit of expanded PICC use," Harnage says. "We feel confident that our success in preventing CLABSIs is a predictable result of our comprehensive approach and dedication to attacking the problem. Zero is achievable, and zero is our goal."

Figure 2-7. Procedure for Central Venous Catheter Dressing Change

Procedure for central venous catheters including non-tunneled central lines (Arrow), peripherally inserted central venous catheters, dialysis catheters, subcutaneous ports, tunneled catheter open ended (Hickman/Broviac) and tunneled catheters valve end (Groshong) type catheters. Routine replacement of CVC dressings are to be completed every 7 days, and every other day for gauze dressings. Exception: dressings are to be changed when visibly damp, loosened, soiled, or when inspection of the site is necessary.

1. Gather supplies: CVC dressing kit, non-sterile gloves, pre-filled normal saline syringe (10ml.) for each lumen, needleless injection cap, dressing retention sheet (Hypafix®) for edges (optional), securement device for PICC, steristrips.

2. Explain procedure to patient. Wash hands and apply clean (non-sterile) gloves.

3. Open packaging to dressing kit, apply mask. Add steri-strips and securement device if needed by opening and dropping onto the sterile field. Have patient turn head away from insertion site throughout procedure, or provide a mask for patient to wear.

4. Remove old dressing being careful NOT to dislodge catheter or touch area around insertion site. Do not use scissors. Discard soiled dressing and gloves.

5. Inspect site for drainage, edema, redness, and area of length of catheter for cording or pain.

6. Apply sterile gloves from kit. Cleanse site and surrounding area with 2% chlorhexadine prep in a back and forth motion using light friction for 30 seconds. Allow to air dry before dressing application.

7. Apply biopatch making 360 degrees skin contact. Do not place on top of catheter.

8. Use steri-strips for excess or non-sutured catheter (as needed). Use securement device for PICC lines.

9. Apply transparent dressing to include entire catheter up to lumen(s) extension. Dressing retention sheet (Hypafix®) to edges if needed (optional).

10. Swab both tip and threads of needleless injection cap vigorously with alcohol (like juicing an orange) for 5-10 seconds before removing. Check for blood return. Apply new needleless injection cap.

11. Flush catheter with 10 ml normal saline using pulsatile, push-pause method.

12. Label new dressing with date, time, initials. For PICC dressing label internal and external length of catheter.

13. Chart on nurses notes dressing change, site condition, arm circumference (10cm. above insertion site for PICC), and external length of catheter. If there are any complications notify MD and chart response.

This protocol serves as a reminder to nurses regarding the appropriate procedure for a central venous catheter dressing change.

Source: Sutter Roseville Medical Center. Used with permission.

Figure 2-8. Central-Line Insertion Data-Collection Tool

Central Line Insertion
Data Collection Tool
NOT PART OF THE PERMANENT RECORD

PATIENT LABEL

Date of Insertion: _____

Unit where CVC placed (select ONLY one):
☐ ICU   ☐ TNI   ☐ NICU   ☐ OR   ☐ IR   ☐ ER   Other Location (specify) _____

Person completing this form (select ONLY one)
☐ Inserter   ☐ RN Assistant/Observer   (PRINTED NAME) _____

Inserted by: ☐ IV Team Staff   ☐ Physician   ☐ PA   ☐ Other _____
Name of person inserting catheter: (PRINTED NAME) _____

Reason for insertion (select ONLY one):
☐ New indication for central line   ☐ Replace malfunctioning central line
☐ Suspected central line-associated infection   ☐ Other (specify) _____

Maximal sterile barrier precautions used:

Person Inserting Catheter			Persons Assisting or at Bedside		Do Not Proceed if Sterile Technique is Not Maintained (unless Emergent Situation)
YES	NO		YES	NO	
☐	☐	Hand hygiene prior to insertion	☐	☐	
☐	☐	Mask or Mask + Eye-protection	☐	☐	
☐	☐	Sterile gown	☐	☐	
☐	☐	Sterile gloves	☐	☐	
☐	☐	Cap	☐	☐	
☐	☐	Large sterile drape			

Skin preparation (check *ALL* that apply):   ☐ Chloraprep   ☐ Alcohol   ☐ Povidone-Iodine
(Chloraprep not recommended for neonates ≤37 weeks gestation)

Was skin prep agent completely dry at time of puncture?:   ☐ Yes   ☐ No

Insertion site: ☐ **Upper** extremity (PICC)   ☐ Subclavian   ☐ Jugular   ☐ Femoral
                 ☐ **Lower** extremity (PICC)   ☐ Umbilical   ☐ Scalp   ☐ Other _____

Antimicrobial coated catheter used: ☐ Yes   ☐ No

Central line catheter type: ☐ PICC (upper extremity)   ☐ Tunneled (NOT dialysis, eg: Broviac™)
                             ☐ Dialysis non-tunneled   ☐ Non-tunneled (NOT dialysis)
                             ☐ Dialysis tunneled   ☐ Umbilical   ☐ Other _____

Number of lumens (Circle one):   1   2   3

Central line is replacing a DC'd line over a guide wire?:   ☐ Yes   ☐ No

Antiseptic ointment applied to site?*   ☐ Yes   ☐ No
    * Note: Use of antiseptic ointment is not an accepted practice

How Secured?:   ☐ Stat-Lok   ☐ Suture

Bio Patch used?:   ☐ Yes   ☐ No   (Note: Bio Patch should be used for every Central Line except Neonates ≤37 weeks gestation)

This form to be completed at the time of the CVC insertion. Once completed, fax to IV Therapy at 878-2111.   rev: 1-12-09

This audit tool is completed for every central venous catheter insertion and is reviewed by infection prevention and control staff.

Source: Sutter Roseville Medical Center. Used with permission.

Ventilator-Associated Pneumonia

VAP is one of the leading causes of morbidity and mortality due to HAIs.[27] The incidence of VAP in mechanically ventilated patients ranges from 4% to 42% and costs around $5,000 per case.[28] VAP can be caused by a number of factors, including aspiration of gastric secretions.[29]

VAP is an infection of the airways that develops more than 48 hours after a patient is intubated.[30] Signs and symptoms of VAP may include the following[31]:
- Two or more serial chest radiographs with at least one of the following:
  - New or progressive *and* persistent infiltrate
  - Consolidation
  - Cavitation
- At least one of the following:
  - Fever of unknown origin
  - Leukopenia or leukocytosis
  - Altered mental status with no known cause in adults $\geq$70 years of age
- At least two of the following:
  - New onset of purulent sputum, change in character of sputum, increased respiratory secretions, or increased suctioning requirements
  - New onset or worsening cough, dyspnea, or tachypnea
  - Rales or bronchial breath sounds
  - Worsening gas exchange, increased oxygen requirements, or increased ventilation demand

According to the IHI, prevention of VAP or prevention of complications of VAP can be accomplished through a ventilator bundle, which includes the following four components[29]:
1. Elevation of the head of the bed to between 30 and 45 degrees
2. Daily "sedation vacation" and daily assessment of readiness to extubate
3. Peptic ulcer disease prophylaxis
4. Deep vein thrombosis prophylaxis (unless contraindicated)

Although most nurses do not prescribe medications, they still need to be aware of indications for pharmacological interventions so they can advocate for their patients when necessary.

Tools for Educating Nursing Staff About the Prevention of VAP

The following tools can help educate staff members about how to prevent VAP:

- **Getting Started Kit: Prevent Ventilator-Associated Pneumonia How-to Guide.** Developed by the IHI. Available at http://www.ihi.org/nr/rdonlyres/d823e3fd-d10b-493e-a6a8-37c767825780/0/vaphowtoguide.doc.
- **PowerPoint Presentation with Facilitator Notes.** Developed by the IHI. Available at http://www.ihi.org/NR/rdonlyres/0F1E9535-3375-4D8D-AFD8-E8923331F68B/0/VAPPresentationwithFacilitorNotesFINAL.ppt.

Common Community-Acquired Infections
Influenza

Influenza is a serious seasonal infection that generally runs from October to May. It causes an average of 36,000 deaths and 226,000 hospitalizations in the United States each year, yet only 42% of health care workers are immunized annually, despite recommendations issued by the CDC.[32] This figure will likely rise with recent outbreaks of H1N1 and other influenza viruses. Influenza vaccination is an important patient-safety issue, because unvaccinated staff can transmit influenza to patients, coworkers, and family members, leading to influenza-related illness and death.[33]

Health care organizations have a responsibility to work aggressively to increase vaccination rates among health care workers.[34] The Joint Commission requires that hospitals, critical access hospitals, and long term care organizations offer influenza vaccinations to licensed independent practitioners and staff. A comprehensive, concerted effort is needed to improve health care worker influenza vaccination rates to optimal levels.[34]

Staff Education

Health care workers are hesitant to be vaccinated for several reasons, and many stem from misperceptions and misunderstandings about the influenza vaccine.[33] Some of the reasons for low immunization rates include the following[33]:

- Concern about side effects
- Perception of low personal risk of illness
- Inconvenience
- Lack of awareness of CDC recommendations
- Fear of needles
- Not believing it makes a difference
- Believing the shot will cause illness

Nurses and other employees can be educated through a variety of channels, such as in-services, employee newsletters, e-mails, posters (*see* Figure 2-9, page 59), and staff intranets (*see* Sidebar 2-2, page 60, for key elements of a successful staff influenza vaccination campaign).[1] Specific interventions that organizations should consider include the following[1]:

- Hold vaccine clinics in easily accessible locations and at varied times.
- Bring the vaccine to employees and licensed independent practitioners via a rolling cart.
- Educate employees and licensed independent practitioners through a variety of methods.
- Remove all costs associated with vaccination.
- Conduct a public health campaign with media coverage.
- Add influenza immunizations to the standard curricula in teaching institutions.

The following are elements to include in any influenza staff and licensed independent practitioner education program[33,34]:

- Injectable influenza vaccine cannot cause influenza.
- Influenza virus is easily transmitted among health care workers and patients, putting already-ill patients at risk for influenza and its complications.
- The CDC recommends an annual vaccination for every health care worker.
- Individuals are generally infectious one to four days before symptom onset, which enables them to spread the virus to others even if they do not yet exhibit symptoms.
- Only around 50% of infected persons will develop symptoms of influenza, yet they can still infect other people.

Remind employees and licensed independent practitioners that although influenza vaccination is the best way to protect against influenza, they can also use other methods to prevent the transmission of influenza[33]:

- Stay at home when sick.
- Sneeze into a tissue or arm/elbow, not into hands.
- Frequently wipe down keyboards, computer mice, and telephones with antibacterial wipes.
- Wash hands or clean them with alcohol-based hand sanitizer frequently.
- Wash hands before eating.
- Avoid contact with people who are sick, except, of course, the patients for whom they are caring.

Figure 2-9. "They Count on You to Get an Influenza Vaccine" Poster

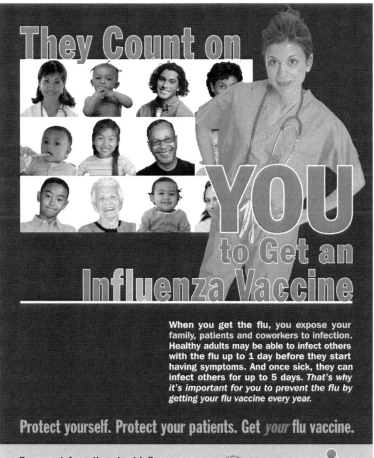

This poster can help educate nursing staff about the potential consequences of not being vaccinated against influenza.

Source: Centers for Disease Control and Prevention. Available at http://www.cdc.gov/flu/freeresources/ (accessed Jun. 9, 2009).

Sidebar 2-2.

Key Elements of a Successful Staff and Licensed Independent Practitioner Influenza Vaccination Campaign

- Inform employees and licensed independent practitioners about the availability of the vaccine and the plan.
- Educate employees and licensed independent practitioners about its importance.
- Make the vaccine convenient.
- Notify employees and licensed independent practitioners regarding the scheduling of the vaccine's administration.
- Keep track of who has been vaccinated so that future educational efforts can be targeted to people who have previously refused vaccination.

Case Study 2-2:
The University of Iowa Hospitals and Clinics' Employee Influenza Campaign

The University of Iowa Hospitals and Clinics (UIHC) began its employee influenza campaign in the early 1990s as part of its employee health program. "The campaign has evolved over the years," says Stephanie Holley, R.N., B.S.N., C.I.C., Quality Management Coordinator, Infection Control Professional, and Nurse Epidemiologist, Program of Hospital Epidemiology, UIHC, Iowa City, Iowa. "We originally provided immunizations at our employee health clinic site, but we've since expanded to add alternative sites. Many of the sites include inpatient units and clinic areas that provide vaccination to all hospital employees in their respective areas using a peer vaccination strategy."

In 2005, UIHC conducted a disaster drill to launch its influenza vaccination campaign. The main objective of the drill was to test its employee mass vaccination/prophylaxis plan by vaccinating as many patient care providers as possible over a six-day period. "The drill scenario occurred during a particularly bad season for influenza," Holley says, "so we set a goal to immunize 70% of our direct patient care providers within that six-day period."

Staff Education. UIHC uses a variety of methods to educate staff about influenza immunization, including the following:

- Notices in the organization's newsletters
- Posters
- Fliers
- Screen savers
- "I got it" stickers
- A list of frequently asked questions (FAQs) on the organization's Web site
- PowerPoint presentations

"We use a multifaceted approach to staff education," Holley says. "Key points about influenza and vaccination are used as screen savers on all of the computers, and notices about vaccination dates, times, and locations are distributed in broadcast e-mails, posters, and newsletters. We have a committee that develops all of our educational materials, posters, and flyers. These are provided to all supervisors and managers for staff distribution. PowerPoint presentations and a list of influenza FAQs are available on our Web site for those who want additional information. We also enlist nurse champions in every area to advocate for health care worker vaccination and to vaccinate everyone on their units, including nurses, physicians, and ancillary personnel. Everyone who receives the vaccination gets an 'I got it' sticker, which lets everyone know that they've been vaccinated."

Holley advises that it is important to involve hospital leadership in any organizationwide employee educational program. "It's important that they be involved," she says. "Leadership needs to be on board in order to send a clear message to staff and to allocate appropriate resources."

Evaluation. In 2007, UIHC switched from a paper to an electronic system for capturing data. "We have over 10,000 employees, so the paper system was quite cumbersome," says Holley. "The new system easily collects real-time data and is able to provide departmental and unit-specific data. It also helps us to capture the people who are declining to be vaccinated. If an employee does not want an influenza vaccination, he or she is asked to formally decline. The system provides a menu of declination reasons for the employee to choose from. The hope is that this will give us information on why employees are declining so we can attempt to address these issues in future vaccination campaigns."

UIHC's current employee influenza immunization rate is 65%. Their goal is 95%. "It's a pretty lofty goal," Holley admits, "but one we think we will eventually reach through teamwork, innovation, and persistence."

Hepatitis B

Every year in the United States, more than 5,000 people die from hepatitis B.[35] Hepatitis B is a disease of the liver that is passed from person to person through unprotected sexual contact, needle sharing, sharing razors, getting a tattoo or body piercing with unsterile equipment, or from mother to baby during birth.[35] Because hepatitis B can be transmitted by blood, nurses are in danger of contracting the disease through needlestick injuries.

Hepatitis B cannot be cured, but it can be prevented by a series of vaccinations. According to the CDC, all health care workers who may be exposed to blood or body fluids should receive a series of three vaccinations, followed by a test for hepatitis B surface antibody (to test for immunity) one to two months after the third dose.

Tools for Educating Staff About Hepatitis B

The following tools can be used to help educate nurses about hepatitis B:
- Brochure: Hepatitis B (HBV). Developed by the APIC (*see* Figure 2-10, page 63).
- The ABCs of Hepatitis. Developed by the CDC (*see* Figure 2-11, page 65).
- Viral Hepatitis: FAQs for Health Professionals. Developed by the CDC. Available at http://www.cdc.gov/hepatitis/HBV/HBVfaq.htm#overview.

Obtaining Diagnostic Specimens

Regardless of whether a patient has been diagnosed with an infection, nurses should be taught to regard all body fluids as potentially infectious.[36] Nurses should also be mindful that failure to decontaminate skin surfaces or needle ports prior to specimen collection can also put patients at risk for infection.

Organizations should educate their nursing staff to always implement standard precautions when obtaining specimens to send to the laboratory. This includes hand hygiene before and after specimen collection, the use of gown (as indicated by standard precautions) and gloves, and appropriate disposal of sharps. Additional measures are specific to certain types of specimens. These are discussed on the following page.

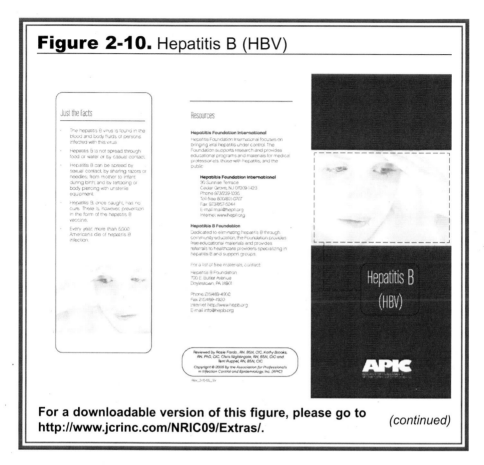

Figure 2-10. Hepatitis B (HBV)

For a downloadable version of this figure, please go to http://www.jcrinc.com/NRIC09/Extras/. *(continued)*

Urine Specimens

Using a needle to aspirate urine through a specimen port of an indwelling urinary catheter puts the nurse at risk for a needlestick injury.[36] Some urinary catheter and drainage system manufacturers sell equipment with needleless access ports. Nursing staff should encourage the people who purchase equipment to look into buying equipment with this type of safety device.

If blood is found in the urine, the nurse is also at risk for exposure to bloodborne pathogens.[36] Additionally, when obtaining a urine sample, splashing can occur, which can pass an infection from the patient to the nurse.[36] In addition to standard precautions, including wearing a mask and face shield, nurses should take the

---

Figure 2-10. Hepatitis B (HBV), *continued*

Hepatitis B

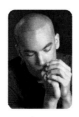

What is Hepatitis B?

The hepatitis B virus infects the liver and can lead to liver failure, liver cancer, and death. Hepatitis B is spread when blood or body fluids from an infected person enters the body of a person who is not infected. The hepatitis B virus is 100 times more contagious than HIV, the virus that causes AIDS.

Are You at Risk?

In 2001 an estimated 78,000 persons in the U.S were infected with hepatitis B. More than 70 percent of those infected are between the ages of 15 and 39.

- Are you sexually active with multiple partners? Or do you have a sexual partner who is at risk for hepatitis B infection?

- Are you a healthcare worker such as a nurse, doctor, physician assistant, nurse practitioner, laboratory technician, emergency room attendant, an employee of an institution for the developmentally disabled, or any other position that exposes you to potentially infected blood or body fluids?

- Do you work in public safety positions such as fire and rescue or law enforcement?

- Are you an immigrant from Asia, Africa, the Amazon Basin in South America, the Pacific Islands, Eastern Europe, or the Middle East?

- Are you a Native American or Alaskan Native?

- Do you live with someone who has hepatitis B?

- Do you practice tattooing or body piercing?

- Do you travel internationally to endemic areas?

- Do you have hemophilia?

- Are you receiving hemodialysis treatments?

- Are you a man who has sex with men?

- Have you ever used intravenous drugs?

If you answered yes to any one of these questions, you are at risk of infection with the hepatitis B virus.

Symptoms

Hepatitis B infects many adults without making them feel sick. You can carry the virus in your body for years without knowing it and unintentionally infect others.

If you do get symptoms, they are like the "flu": you lose your appetite, feel extremely tired, have stomach cramps, and throw up. If you are more seriously ill, your skin and eyes may turn yellow and you may need to be admitted to the hospital.

Acute hepatitis: Lasts no longer than 6 months, after which you are no longer infectious.

Chronic hepatitis: Lasts longer than 6 months and you remain infectious.

How can I protect myself?

The only way to protect yourself from infection is by getting vaccinated (a three-shot series). If you are at risk, talk with your doctor today about getting the hepatitis B vaccination.

This brochure can help educate nurses about risk factors for hepatitis B and methods of prevention.

Source: Association for Professionals in Infection Control and Epidemiology. Used with permission.

---

following steps to prevent infection when obtaining urine samples from indwelling urinary catheters[36,37]:

- Use aseptic technique.
- Wipe the sampling port with an alcohol swab before and after specimen collection.
- Unclamp the catheter tubing after obtaining the sample to prevent the backflow of urine, which may cause a UTI.
- Monitor patient for signs of UTI. Any breach in the closed system, such as taking a urine sample, can increase the patient's risk for UTI.

Figure 2-11. The ABCs of Hepatitis

The ABCs of Hepatitis

	HEPATITIS A is caused by the hepatitis A virus (HAV)	**HEPATITIS B** is caused by the hepatitis B virus (HBV)	**HEPATITIS C** is caused by the hepatitis C virus (HCV)
Statistics	• Estimated 32,000 new infections in 2006	• Estimated 46,000 new infections in 2006 • Estimated 800,000–1.4 million people with chronic HBV infection	• Estimated 19,000 new infections in 2006 • Estimated 3.2 million people with chronic HCV infection
Routes of Transmission	Ingestion of fecal matter, even in microscopic amounts, from: • Close person-to-person contact with an infected person • Sexual contact with an infected person • Ingestion of contaminated food or drinks	Contact with infectious blood, semen, and other body fluids, primarily through: • Birth to an infected mother • Sexual contact with an infected person • Sharing of contaminated needles, syringes or other injection drug equipment • Needlesticks or other sharp instrument injuries	Contact with blood of an infected person, primarily through: • Sharing of contaminated needles, syringes, or other injection drug equipment Less commonly through: • Sexual contact with an infected person • Birth to an infected mother • Needlestick or other sharp instrument injuries
Persons at Risk	• Travelers to regions with intermediate or high rates of hepatitis A • Sex contacts of infected persons • Household members or caregivers of infected persons • Men who have sex with men • Users of certain illegal drugs (injection and non-injection) • Persons with clotting-factor disorders	• Infants born to infected mothers • Sex partners of infected persons • Persons with multiple sex partners • Persons with a sexually transmitted disease (STD) • Men who have sex with men • Injection drug users • Household contacts of infected persons • Healthcare and public safety workers exposed to blood on the job • Hemodialysis patients • Residents and staff of facilities for developmentally disabled persons • Travelers to regions with intermediate or high rates of hepatitis B (HBsAg prevalence of ≥2%)	• Current or former injection drug users • Recipients of clotting factor concentrates before 1987 • Recipients of blood transfusions or donated organs before July 1992 • Long-term hemodialysis patients • Persons with known exposures to HCV (e.g., healthcare workers after needlesticks, recipients of blood or organs from a donor who later tested positive for HCV) • HIV-infected persons • Infants born to infected mothers
Incubation Period	15 to 50 days (average: 28 days)	45 to 160 days (average: 120 days)	14 to 180 days (average: 45 days)
Symptoms of Acute Infection	Symptoms of all types of viral hepatitis are similar and can include one or more of the following: • Fever • Fatigue • Loss of appetite • Nausea • Vomiting • Abdominal pain • Clay-colored bowel movements • Joint pain • Jaundice		
Likelihood of Symptomatic Acute Infection	• < 10% of children < 6 years have jaundice • 40%–50% of children age 6–14 years have jaundice • 70%–80% of persons > 14 years have jaundice	• < 1% of infants < 1 year develop symptoms • 5%–15% of children age 1-5 years develop symptoms • 30%–50% of persons > 5 years develop symptoms Note: Symptoms appear in 5%–15% of newly infected adults who are immunosuppressed	• 20%–30% of newly infected persons develop symptoms of acute disease
Potential for Chronic Infection	None	• Among unimmunized persons, chronic infection occurs in >90% of infants, 25%–50% of children aged 1–5 years, and 6%–10% of older children and adults	• 75%–85% of newly infected persons develop chronic infection • 15%–20% of newly infected persons clear the virus
Severity	Most persons with acute disease recover with no lasting liver damage; rarely fatal	• Most persons with acute disease recover with no lasting liver damage; acute illness is rarely fatal • 15%–25% of chronically infected persons develop chronic liver disease, including cirrhosis, liver failure, or liver cancer • Estimated 2,000–4,000 persons in the United States die from HBV-related illness per year	• Acute illness is uncommon. Those who do develop acute illness recover with no lasting liver damage. • 60%–70% of chronically infected persons develop chronic liver disease • 5%–20% develop cirrhosis over a period of 20–30 years • 1%–5% will die from cirrhosis or liver cancer • Estimated 8,000–10,000 persons in the United States die from HCV-related illness per year
Serologic Tests	• IgM anti-HAV is recommended for diagnosing acute disease • Screening for past infection is generally not recommended	• HBsAg is recommended for screening most populations • See guidelines for appropriate follow-up testing as indicated in screening recommendations • See guidelines for identifying and testing high-risk populations	• Screening assay (EIA or CIA) for anti-HCV • Verification by an additional more specific assay (e.g., RIBA for anti-HCV) or nucleic acid testing for HCV RNA

For a downloadable version of this figure, please go to Http://www.jcrinc.com/NRIC09/Extras/. *(continued)*

Figure 2-11. The ABCs of Hepatitis, *continued*

	HEPATITIS A	HEPATITIS B	HEPATITIS C
Treatment	• No medication available • Best addressed through supportive treatment	• Acute: No medication available; best addressed through supportive treatment • Chronic: Regular monitoring for signs of liver disease progression; some patients are treated with antiviral drugs	• Acute: Antivirals and supportive treatment • Chronic: Regular monitoring for signs of liver disease progression; some patients are treated with antiviral drugs
Vaccination Recommendations	Hepatitis A vaccine is recommended for: • All children at age 1 year • Travelers to regions with intermediate or high rates of hepatitis A • Men who have sex with men • Users of certain illegal drugs (injection and non-injection) • Persons with clotting-factor disorders • Persons who work with HAV-infected primates or with HAV in a research laboratory • Persons with chronic liver disease, including HBV- and HCV-infected persons with chronic liver disease • Anyone else seeking long-term protection	Hepatitis B vaccine is recommended for: • All infants within 12 hours of birth • Older children who have not previously been vaccinated • Sex partners of infected persons • Persons with multiple sex partners • Persons seeking evaluation or treatment for an STD • Men who have sex with men • Injection drug users • Household contacts of infected persons • Healthcare and public safety workers exposed to blood on the job • Persons with chronic liver disease, including HCV-infected persons with chronic liver disease • Persons with HIV infection • Persons with end-stage renal disease, including predialysis, hemodialysis, peritoneal dialysis, and home dialysis patients • Residents and staff of facilities for developmentally disabled persons • Travelers to regions with intermediate or high rates of hepatitis B (HBsAg prevalence of ≥2%) • Anyone else seeking long-term protection	There is no hepatitis C vaccine.
Vaccination Schedule	2 doses given 6 months apart	• Infants and children: 3 to 4 doses given over a 6- to 18-month period depending on vaccine type and schedule • Adults: 3 doses given over a 6-month period	No vaccine available
Testing Recommendations	Pre-vaccination testing (anti-HAV) can be considered for populations that have expected high rates of prior HAV infection, such as: • Adults born in, or who lived for extensive periods in, regions with intermediate or high rates of hepatitis A • Older adolescents and adults of certain races/ethnicities (American Indians, Alaska Natives, Hispanics) • Injection drug users Postvaccination testing is not recommended because of the high rate of vaccine response.	Testing for HBsAg (and additional markers as needed) is recommended for: • Pregnant women • Persons born in regions with intermediate or high rates of hepatitis B (HBsAg prevalence of ≥2%) • U.S.–born persons not vaccinated as infants whose parents were born in regions with high rates of hepatitis B (HBsAg prevalence of ≥ 8%) • Infants born to HBsAg-positive mothers • Household, needle-sharing, or sex contacts of HBsAg-positive persons • Men who have sex with men • Injection drug users • Patients with elevated liver enzymes (ALT/AST) of unknown etiology • Hemodialysis patients • Persons needing immunosuppressive or cytotoxic therapy • HIV-infected persons • Sources of blood or body fluids involved in potential HBV exposures (e.g., needlesticks) • Donors of blood, plasma, organs, tissues, or semen	Testing is recommended for: • Current or former injection drug users • Recipients of clotting factor concentrates before 1987 • Recipients of blood transfusions or donated organs before July 1992 • Long-term hemodialysis patients • Persons with known exposures to HCV (e.g., healthcare workers after needlesticks, recipients of blood or organs from a donor who later tested positive for HCV) • HIV-infected persons • Children born to infected mothers (do not test before age 18 mos.) • Patients with signs or symptoms of liver disease (e.g., abnormal liver enzyme tests) • Donors of blood, plasma, organs, tissues, or semen

DEPARTMENT OF HEALTH & HUMAN SERVICES
Centers for Disease Control and Prevention

Division of Viral Hepatitis

CDC

This handout provides a comparison of hepatitis A, hepatitis B, and hepatitis C.

Source: Centers for Disease Control and Prevention. Available at http://www.cdc.gov/hepatitis/Resources/Professionals/PDFs/ABCTable.pdf (accessed Dec. 2, 2009).

Blood Samples

Drawing blood samples puts the nurse or the phlebotomist at risk for contracting bloodborne pathogens via needlestick injury or direct contact with a patient's blood. The wound from the needlestick also becomes a portal for infectious agents to enter the patient. In addition to standard precautions, including wearing a mask and face shield, nurses or phlebotomists should take the following steps to prevent infection when obtaining blood samples[38–40]:

- If drawing blood through a central venous catheter, use aseptic technique.
- Clean the area or catheter hub with an alcohol swab or other agent per organizational protocol; allow the area to air dry.
- Do not palpate the venipuncture site after it has been cleaned, even if wearing sterile gloves.
- To decrease the risk of needlestick injury, do not hold specimen containers in your hand when transferring blood from the syringe to a culture container.
- If blood does not flow easily from the syringe to the culture container, do not force it. This may cause blood spatter.
- Use the clean technique for phlebotomy.

Nasal Swabs

Nasal swabs are frequently used to detect MRSA or to diagnose respiratory viruses or infections.[41] Nasal secretions that contain infectious agents can transmit infection from the patient to the nurse if proper procedures are not followed. In addition to standard precautions, nurses should take the following steps to prevent cross-contamination of specimens or false positive results when obtaining nasal swabs[41]:

- Do not use swab packages that have been opened or swabs that have expired.
- Do not touch the swab to any surface except the nasal passage.
- Be careful to not contaminate the swab when placing it in the culture medium.

Stool Specimens

Stool specimens are collected to detect the presence of occult blood for colorectal cancer screening or to detect organisms, such as *C. difficile,* and for diagnosing other infections. In addition to standard precautions, the following steps can be taken to help prevent cross-contamination from the patient to the nurse or to prevent contamination of the specimen[42]:

- Use a clinically clean receptacle for collecting the specimen.
- Use the spoon provided in the sample kit to transfer the specimen to the container.
- Avoid specimens that have been contaminated with urine.

Sputum Specimens

Sputum specimens can be used to diagnose lung cancer or infections, such as tuberculosis.[43] In addition to standard precautions, the following steps can be taken to help prevent cross-contamination from the patient to the nurse or to prevent introducing a new infection to the patient[43]:

- Step away from the patient while he or she is expectorating the sample into the receptacle.
- Use aseptic technique if obtaining a specimen from an indwelling tracheal cannula.

Administering Intramuscular or Intravenous Medications

According to the CDC, recent hepatitis B and hepatitis C outbreaks may have been avoided if staff members were properly educated about and adhered to the basic principles of infection prevention and control and aseptic technique.[44] Two primary breaches in infection prevention and control practices contributed to the recent outbreaks. These breaches were (1) reinsertion of used needles into multiple-dose vials or solution containers and (2) use of a single needle/syringe to administer IV medications to multiple patients.[44] To ensure that nurses are appropriately educated about recommended practices, principles of infection prevention and control and aseptic technique should be included in all training programs.[44]

To assist organizations with education about infection prevention and control practices during intramuscular or IV medication administration, the CDC developed the following safe-injection practices[44]:

- Use aseptic technique to avoid contamination of sterile injection equipment.
- Do not administer medications from a syringe to multiple patients, even if the needle or cannula on the syringe is changed. Needles, cannulas, and syringes are sterile, single-use items; they should not be reused for another patient or to access a medication or solution that might be used for a subsequent patient.
- Use fluid infusion and administration sets (that is, intravenous bags, tubing, and connectors) for one patient only, and dispose of them appropriately after use. Consider a syringe or needle/cannula contaminated once it has been used to enter or to connect to a patient's intravenous infusion bag or administration set.
- Use single-dose vials for parenteral medications whenever possible.
- Do not administer medications from single-dose vials or ampuls to multiple patients or combine leftover contents for later use.

- If multidose vials must be used, the needle or cannula and syringe used to access the multidose vial must be sterile. A new needle or cannula and syringe must be used each time.
- Do not keep multidose vials in the immediate patient treatment area, and store them in accordance with the manufacturer's recommendations; discard if sterility is compromised or questionable.
- Do not use bags or bottles of intravenous solution as a common source of supply for multiple patients.
- For lumbar puncture procedures, wear a surgical mask when placing a catheter or injecting material into the spinal canal or subdural space (that is, during myelograms, lumbar puncture, and spinal or epidural anesthesia).
- Adhere to federal and state requirements for protection of healthcare personnel from exposure to bloodborne pathogens.

Preventing Cross-Contamination When Using Charts/Computers

Objects in patient care areas, such as patient charts and computer equipment, can easily be contaminated by nurses or other health care personnel. Patient charts are handled by multiple staff and licensed independent practitioners. They are also frequently taken into patient rooms, even for those patients who are on isolation precautions, and sometimes set on the patient's bed—contrary to recommended practices.[45] These actions increase the risk for cross-contamination by way of the health care worker's hands and should be discouraged during educational programs for nurses and other patient care staff.[45]

Because disinfection of patient charts may not be practical, the best solution for prevention of cross-contamination via patient charts is appropriate hand hygiene after patient care and before writing in the patient chart.[46] Hand hygiene after contact with a potentially contaminated chart can also help reduce the transmission of infection.[46]

Because computers have become commonplace in patient care areas, nurses should be taught that they are also potential reservoirs for infectious agents.[47] In addition, computer keyboards are difficult to disinfect and are not always disinfected on a routine basis.[48,49] Nurses should be made aware that the risk of cross-contamination by way of computer equipment could be greatly reduced or eliminated by appropriate hand hygiene. Additionally, keyboards that are used in patient care

What Would You Do?

A charge nurse on a medical/surgical unit approaches a computer and notices that the keyboard is visibly soiled. She goes to a supply closet to get some disinfectant wipes to clean the keys. When she returns, she notes that a nurse is sitting at the computer using the soiled keyboard. As she watches, the nurse picks up a patient chart, makes a note, and then returns to the keyboard. When she is finished typing, the nurse walks away from the computer and heads for one of the patient rooms.

In this scenario, infection could be spread from the keyboard to the nurse's hands, from the nurse's hands to the patient chart, or from the patient chart to the keyboard. It could also be spread to the patient if the nurse fails to perform hand hygiene before caring for the next patient.

Because objects in patient care or common areas can easily become contaminated, and because they are handled by patient care staff, this scenario raises the opportunity to educate all patient care staff about preventing cross-contamination when using charts or computers. Education could be done in a variety of ways, such as informally at shift change, via a staff memo, or at an in-service for patient care staff.

areas should be disinfected daily and when visibly soiled.[49] Keyboard covers or water-resistant keyboards can facilitate disinfection procedures.[48]

Monitoring and Maintaining Patient Hygiene

Poor hygiene practices can lead to infection. Nurses have a responsibility to ensure that their patients are assisted with activities that contribute to good hygiene, such as bathing, hand hygiene, oral care, catheter care, and incontinence management.[50] If these activities are performed by a nursing assistant (NA) or a patient care technician (PCT), the nurse is responsible for overseeing the work of the NA or PCT. Therefore, nurses should be educated not only about methods for maintaining patient hygiene but also about following up to see that the work has been done correctly. For example, the nurse might observe the NA or the PCT providing oral care to assess for appropriate technique.

Nurses can also assist patients in maintaining good hygiene by monitoring patient hygiene practices and acting on educational opportunities. For example, if a nurse sees a patient getting ready for a meal, he or she might offer to assist the patient with hand hygiene and use that opportunity to remind the patient that hand hygiene should be done after toileting and before meals.

Health Care–Associated Infection Compendium

A Compendium of Strategies to Prevent Healthcare-Associated Infections in Acute Care Hospitals is a collaborative effort between The Joint Commission, the Society for Healthcare Epidemiology in America, APIC, the Infectious Diseases Society of America, and the American Hospital Association. It is implementation-focused and unique in that it highlights a set of basic HAI prevention strategies and includes special approaches for use in locations and/or populations within the hospital.[51] It also includes proposed performance measures for internal quality improvement efforts.[51]

The HAI compendium focuses on the following six HAI categories:
- SSIs
- CLABSIs
- CAUTIs
- VAP
- *C. diff*
- MRSA

Each HAI category follows the same format and includes a purpose, rationale and statements of concern, detection strategies, prevention strategies, recommendations for implementing prevention and monitoring strategies, and performance measures.

Despite good intentions, HAIs occur in U.S. hospitals every day, resulting in serious illness and death.[52] This compendium of strategies to prevent HAIs was created to provide a concise, evidence-based resource containing practical recommendations for acute care hospitals.[52] The compendium can be downloaded at no cost at http://www.journals.uchicago.edu/toc/iche/2008/29/s1.

References

1. The Joint Commission: *The Joint Commission Guide to Staff Education,* 2nd ed. Oakbrook Terrace, IL: Joint Commission Resources, 2008.

2. Joint Commission Resources: Health care–associated infections: Safeguards for infection-free care. *The Source* 6:4–5, 10, Feb. 2008.

3. Suchitra J.G., Devi N.L.: Impact of education on knowledge, attitudes and practices among various categories of health care workers on nosocomial infections. *Indian J Med Microbiol* 25:181–187, Jul. 2007.

4. Beggs C.B., et al.: The influence of nurse cohorting on hand hygiene effectiveness. *Am J Infect Control* 34:621–626, Dec. 2006.

5. Centers for Disease Control and Prevention: *Guideline for Hand Hygiene in Health-Care Settings.* Oct. 25, 2002. http://www.cdc.gov/mmwr/preview/mmwrhtml/rr5116a1.htm (accessed Jan. 5, 2009).

6. Joint Commission Resources: Preventing surgical site infections. *Joint Commission Perspectives on Patient Safety* 8:8–9, 11, Sep. 2008.

7. Centers for Disease Control and Prevention, National Center for Health Statistics Vital and Health Statistics: *Detailed Diagnoses and Procedures National Hospital Discharge Survey 1994.* Hyattsville, MD: Department of Health and Human Services, 1997.

8. Institute for Health Improvement: *Getting Started Kit: Prevent Surgical Site Infection, How-to Guide.* http://www.ihi.org/nr/rdonlyres/c54b5133-f4bb-4360-a3e4-2952c08c9b59/0/ssihowtoguide.doc (accessed Jan. 15, 2009).

9. Saint Agnes Medical Center: *Preparing for Surgery.* http://www.samc.com/UMAP/UserPageObjects/Brochure_PrepSurgery.pdf (accessed Jun. 18, 2009).

10. The Joint Commission: Update: The Joint Commission's position on steam sterilization. *Joint Commission Perspectives* 29: 8, 11, July 2009.

11. Odom-Forren J.: Preventing surgical site infections. *Nursing* 36:59–63, Jun. 2006.

12. Anderson D.J., et al.: *Strategies to Prevent Surgical Site Infections in Acute Care Hospitals.* Oct. 2008. http://www.journals.uchicago.edu/doi/full/10.1086/591064 (accessed Jun. 18, 2009).

13. Centers for Disease Control and Prevention: *Management of Multidrug-Resistant Organisms in Healthcare Settings, 2006.* http://www.cdc.gov/ncidod/dhqp/pdf/ar/MDROGuideline2006.pdf (accessed Mar. 30, 2009).

14. Joint Commission Resources: Battling "superbugs" in the environment of care: New CDC guidelines include recommendations for environmental services. *Environment of Care News* 10:1–4, Feb. 2007.

15. Archibald L.K., Banerjee S.N., Jarvis W.R.: Secular trends in hospital-acquired *Clostridium difficile* disease in the United States, 1987–2001. *J Infect Dis* 189(9):1585–1589, 2004.

16. McDonald L.C., Owings M., Jernigan D.B.: *Clostridium difficile* infection in patients discharged from U.S. short-stay hospitals, 1996–2003. *Emerg Infect Dis* 12(3): Internet serial, Oct. 2005. http://www.cdc.gov/ncidod/EID/vol12no03/pdfs/05-1064.pdf (accessed Jan. 15, 2009).

17. McGoldrick M., Rhinehart E.: Managing multidrug-resistant organisms in home care and hospice. *Home Healthc Nurse* 25:580–586, Oct. 2007.

18. Joint Commission Resources: 5 Million Lives campaign: Reducing methicillin-resistant *Staphylococcus aureus* (MRSA) infections. *Jt Comm J Qual Patient* Saf 33:726–731, Dec. 2007.

19. Yamamoto L.: Listen up MRSA: The bug stops here. *Nursing* 37:51–55, quiz 55–56, Dec. 2007.

20. Joint Commission Resources: The top five: New lookouts and outlooks on the vancomycin resistance front. *The Source* 3:11, Dec. 2001.

21. Centers for Disease Control and Prevention: *Multiple-Drug Resistant Enterococci: The Nature of the Problem and an Agenda for the Future.* Apr.–Jun. 1998. http://www.cdc.gov/ncidod/ eid/vol4no2/HUYCKE.HTM (accessed Jun. 18, 2009).

22. Centers for Disease Control and Prevention: *Guideline for Prevention of Catheter-Associated Urinary Tract Infections.* Feb. 1981. http://www.cdc.gov/ncidod/dhqp/gl_catheter_assoc.html (accessed Jan. 21, 2009).

23. Institute for Healthcare Improvement: *Getting Started Kit: Prevent Central Line Infections How-to Guide.* http://www.ihi.org/nr/rdonlyres/0ad706aa-0e76-457b-a4b0-78c31a5172d8/ 0/centrallineinfectionshowtoguide.doc (accessed Jan. 21, 2009).

24. Polzien G.: Home infusion therapy. First things first: The patient and the prevention of central catheter infections. *Home Healthc Nurse* 24:681–684, Nov.–Dec. 2006.

25. Harnage S.A.: Achieving zero catheter-related bloodstream infections: 15 months success in a community-based medical center. *J Vasc Access* 12:218–224, Dec. 2007.

26. Harnage S.A.: Frontline fame: A PICC team ends CRBSIs. *RN* 71:34–36, 38–39, May 2008.

27. Kaynar A.M., et al.: Attitudes of respiratory therapists and nurses about measures to prevent ventilator-associated pneumonia: A multicenter, cross-sectional survey study. *Respir Care* 52:1687–1694, Dec. 2007.

28. Roy G.L.: Interventions by critical care nurses reduce VAP. *Dynamics* 18:28–31, quiz 32–33, Fall 2007.

29. Institute for Healthcare Improvement: *What You Need to Know About Ventilator-Associated Pneumonia (VAP): A Fact Sheet for Patients and Their Family Members.* http://www.ihi.org/ NR/rdonlyres/818C1992-F318-4DBD-AE54-B45BCD3AD7DB/0/ VentilatorAssociatedPneumoniaPatandFamSheet.pdf (accessed Jan. 15, 2009).

30. Institute for Healthcare Improvement: *Implement the Ventilator Bundle.* http://www.ihi.org/ IHI/Topics/CriticalCare/IntensiveCare/Changes/ImplementtheVentilatorBundle.htm (accessed Jun. 18, 2009).

31. Klompas M., Platt R.: *Ventilator-Associated Pneumonia Rates: The Wrong Quality Measure.* Dec. 2007. http://www.acphospitalist.org/archives/2007/12/vap_qm.htm (accessed Jun. 18, 2009).

32. Association for Professionals in Infection Control and Epidemiology: *APIC Position Paper: Influenza Immunization of Healthcare Personnel.* http://www.apic.org/AM/Template.cfm? Section=Home1&TEMPLATE=/CM/ContentDisplay.cfm&CONTENTFILEID=11049 (accessed Jan. 2, 2009).

33. U.S. Department of Veterans Affairs: *Influenza/Flu—Improving Health Care Worker Vaccination Rates.* http://www.publichealth.va.gov/flu/flu_hcw.htm (accessed Jan. 2, 2009).

34. National Foundation for Infectious Diseases: *Improving Influenza Vaccination Rates in Health Care Workers.* http://www.nfid.org/pdf/publications/hcwmonograph.pdf (accessed Jan. 2, 2009).

35. Association for Professionals in Infection Control: *Hepatitis B (HBV).* Mar. 10, 2005. http://www.apic.org/AM/Template.cfm?Section=Search&section=Brochures&template=/CM/ContentDisplay.cfm&ContentFileID=8998 (accessed Apr. 8, 2009).

36. Roodhouse A., Wellsted A.: Safety in urine sampling: Maintaining an infection-free environment. *Br J Nurs* 15:870–872, Sep. 2006.

37. Higgins D.: Specimen collection: Obtaining a catheter specimen of urine. *Nurs Times* 104:26–27, May 2008.

38. Moureau N.L.: Drawing blood through a central venous catheter. *Nursing* 34:28, Feb. 2004.

39. Rushing J.: Drawing blood culture specimens for reliable results. *Nursing* 34:20, Dec. 2004.

40. Rushing J.: Drawing blood with vacuum tubes. *Nursing* 34:26, Jan. 2004.

41. Higgins D.: Specimen collection: Collecting a stool specimen. *Nurs Times* 104:22–23, May 2008.

42. Higgins D.: Specimen collection: Obtaining a catheter specimen of urine. *Nurs Times* 104:26–27, May 2008.

43. Specimen collection: Obtaining a sputum sample. *Nurs Times* 104:26–27, May 2008.

44. Centers for Disease Control and Prevention: *Safe Injection Practices to Prevent Transmission of Infections to Patients.* Updated Mar. 28, 2008. http://www.cdc.gov/ncidod/dhqp/injectionSafetyPractices.html (accessed Apr. 6, 2009).

45. Bebbington A., et al.: Patients' case-notes: Look but don't touch. *J Hosp Infect* 55:299–301, Dec. 2003.

46. Panhotra B.R., Saxena A.K., Al-Mulhim A.S.: Contamination of patients' files in intensive care units: An indication of strict handwashing after entering case notes. *Am J Infect Control* 33:398–401, Sep. 2005.

47. Neely A.N., et al.: Computer equipment used in patient care within a multihospital system: Recommendations for cleaning and disinfection. *Am J Infect Control* 33:233–237, May 2005.

48. Schultz M., et al.: Bacterial contamination of computer keyboards in a teaching hospital. *Infect Control Hosp Epidemiol* 24:302–303, Apr. 2003.

49. Rutala W.A., et al.: Bacterial contamination of keyboards: Efficacy and functional impact of disinfectants. *Infect Control Hosp Epidemiol* 27:372–377, Apr. 2006.

50. McGuckin M., Shubin A., Hujcs M.: Interventional patient hygiene model: Infection control and nursing share responsibility for patient safety. *Am J Infect Control* 36:59–62, Feb. 2008.

51. Yokoe D.S., et al.: Executive Summary: *A Compendium of Strategies to Prevent Healthcare-Associated Infections in Acute Care Hospitals.* Oct. 2008. http://www.journals.uchicago.edu/doi/full/10.1086/591060 (accessed Jun. 18, 2009).

52. Yokoe D.S., Classen D.: *Improving Patient Safety Through Infection Control: A New Healthcare Imperative.* Oct. 2008.

Chapter 3

Partnering with Other Disciplines to Help Prevent and Control Infections

To improve infection prevention and control efforts, systemwide action on a broad range of fronts is necessary to identify and to manage actual and potential risks.[1] This requires actions in staff and patient education, performance improvement, environmental safety, and risk management, and it embraces all health care disciplines.[1] Table 3-1, page 76, provides a quick reference for the role nurse's play in interacting with many disciplines throughout an organization.

Disease-causing organisms can breed in cooling towers, ice machines, humidifiers, and drains. They are found in elevator shafts, ceiling tiles, and central vacuum systems. Staff can transmit organisms via their hands. Equipment that is not properly cleaned can pass organisms from one patient to another. So it is essential that all staff, direct care providers, and ancillary personnel be educated about their roles in reducing or preventing the spread of infection.[2]

Nurses Working with Infection Preventionists

Many health care organizations employ infection preventionists (IPs) whose sole purpose is to prevent infections and to control outbreaks. Because nurses are on the front line of patient care, they are perfectly positioned to work collaboratively with IPs in infection prevention and control efforts and initiatives. One option is to have nurses providing direct patient care serve as members of the organization's infection prevention and control committee. As committee members, nurses can participate in the review of literature for best practices, collaborate in the development of infection prevention and control protocols for nurses based on care practices, interview nurses about current infection prevention and control practices, and conduct infection control tracers. These nurses can act as liaisons between infection prevention and control staff and unit-based nurses.

Table 3-1. Common Interactions Related to IP&C Between Nurses and Other Disciplines

Nurses Working with...	Interactions
Infection preventionists	Collaborate on IP&C efforts and initiatives; IP&C committee; IP unit liaison; monitor changes in practice or equipment and alert IP; assist with data collection; and help with unit staff education
Physicians and other licensed independent practitioners	Conduct multidisciplinary unit-based initiatives to prevent specific types of infection; and identify who is responsible for each step of a process
Other patient care staff	Ensure protocols for hand hygiene, contact precautions, patient movement while under contact precautions, and urinary catheter care are followed; make sure medication lists are up-to-date; administer medications in a timely manner and document patient response to treatment; develop evidence-based protocols for patients on ventilators; ensure PCTs, CNAs, and nursing students are adequately trained in infection prevention and control practices
Nonclinical staff	Assure that nonclinical staff understand role in infection prevention; ensure that protocols for hand hygiene, standard precautions, and contact precautions are being followed; alert staff of breaches in infection prevention and control protocols; check that gowns and gloves are readily available; help educate and train staff

Key: CNA: certified nursing assistant; IP: infection preventionist; IP&C: infection prevention and control; PCT: patient care technician

Although all nurses will not be able to participate on the infection prevention committee, they may have other opportunities to take active roles in the organization's infection prevention program. Numerous health care facilities have developed programs where an infection prevention liaison is stationed on each nursing unit. One of the primary roles of an infection prevention liaison is to assist in early detection of outbreaks on the unit.[3] Other roles include helping the IP increase awareness of infection prevention and control issues on the unit, alerting the IP to changes in practice or equipment, assisting with data collection, acting as an opinion leader, and helping with staff education on the unit.[3]

Collaboration between unit staff and the IP on the development of unit-based infection prevention efforts, such as the elimination of central line–associated bloodstream infections (CLABSIs), is a powerful infection prevention initiative. And it takes advantage of the staff's familiarity with patient care practices on the unit as well as their insights as practices are changed to improve patient outcomes. In some organizations, nurses are employed as IPs. Many devote all their time to infection prevention and control initiatives. Others work part time as direct care providers so they can stay current on patient care practices and see the results of practice changes.

Compliance monitoring is another way in which nurses and IPs can work together to prevent and to control infections. Holding peers and other health care providers accountable for compliance with infection prevention practices is important, and caregivers should imbed these practices into their daily routines. For example, if one nurse observes another nurse failing to perform hand hygiene between patients, he or she has the opportunity and the obligation to point out the breech. In a culture that uses errors as an opportunity for learning, the nurse who has been reminded to perform hand hygiene would accept the constructive criticism gracefully.

Developing Sustainable Infection Prevention and Control Practices

Infection prevention and control programs need to be well managed to be effective. Therefore, organizational leadership should assign responsibility for development and management of the program to one or more people. Depending on the size of the facility and facility resources, the program manager may be an employee, a contractor, or a consultant.[4]

Planning

After a program leader has been identified, the work of planning the infection prevention and control program can begin by gathering individuals with expertise in infection prevention and control, facilities management, and other key services who can perform a risk assessment and put in place infection prevention and control strategies, plans, and activities. The infection prevention and control team may want to consult with community leaders and other outside infection prevention and control experts who can provide important information about the organization's population and associated health risks.[4]

The results of the organization's infection risk assessment should be prioritized, ideally in order of level of probability and potential for harm. The facility can then set goals for reducing or eliminating the risks of the infections that pose the most threat to patients and the community. These goals should lead to focused activities, based on relevant professional guidelines and sound scientific practices.[4]

Planning should include the following[4]:
- Identification of the individual(s) responsible for the infection prevention and control program
- Allocation of needed resources for the infection prevention and control program
- Identification of risks for acquiring and transmitting infections
- Development of goals to minimize infection transmission, based on the organization's identified risks
- Development of a written infection prevention and control plan describing activities, including surveillance, intended to minimize, to reduce, or to eliminate the risk of infection
- A process, preferably written, for communicating responsibilities about preventing and controlling infection to licensed independent practitioners, staff, visitors, patients, and families
- A written response plan for the influx of potentially infectious patients
- A method for communicating critical information to licensed independent practitioners and staff about emerging infections that could cause an influx of potentially infectious patients

Implementation

The activities of infection prevention and control should be practical and should involve collaboration between departments and staff. Everyone who works in the facility should have a role and hold each other accountable. Important infection prevention and control information should be available to staff and patients. Standard and transmission-based precautions should be used, and any outbreak of infection within the hospital should be investigated.[4]

All infection prevention and control programs should include a surveillance element in which infection data are collected, analyzed, monitored, and acted upon to prevent future infections and to halt outbreaks when they occur.

Implementation should include the following[4]:
- Implementation of the organizational infection prevention and control plan
- Communication of responsibilities for preventing and controlling infection to licensed independent practitioners, staff, visitors, patients, and families
- Reporting infection surveillance, prevention, and control information to the appropriate organizational staff and leaders
- Strategies to reduce the risk of infections associated with medical equipment, devices, and supplies
- Strategies to prevent the transmission of infectious disease among patients, licensed independent practitioners, staff, and visitors
- An influenza vaccination program for licensed independent practitioners and staff that includes the following:
  - Vaccine at no cost
  - Education about influenza vaccine; nonvaccine prevention and control measures; and the diagnosis, transmission, and impact of influenza

Evaluation

Evaluation and improvement of the hospital's infection prevention and control activities are important steps in the organization's efforts to control and to prevent infection. Infection prevention and control practices need to become routine parts of the care, treatment, and services the facility provides to patients. They expect and deserve hygienic and safe care at all times. Continuous review of the goals, activities, and outcomes of the hospital's program are therefore followed by improvement activities that are effective and realistic in expectation.[4]

Evaluation should include the following[4]:
- Assessment of the effectiveness of the infection prevention and control plan annually and whenever risks significantly change

- Communication of evaluation results, at least annually, to the individuals or interdisciplinary group that manages the patient safety program

Case Study 3-1:
Children's Hospital of Philadelphia

Health care–associated infections (HAIs) result in significant morbidity and mortality. In the United States, 1.7 million patients annually acquire infections while hospitalized for other conditions.[1] HAIs result in 99,000 deaths[1] annually, at an approximate cost of $5 billion.[2] Almost one third of these deaths is associated with catheter-associated bloodstream infections in adult and pediatric patients hospitalized in nonintensive care settings.[1]

Established in 1855, the Children's Hospital of Philadelphia is one of the leading pediatric hospitals and research facilities in the world. Despite the dedicated care that it provides to patients and their families, it found itself confronted with an increase in the incidence of CLABSIs. To combat this issue, in August 2008, the nursing leadership group of 8 South, the patient care unit dedicated to endocrine and digestive disorders, developed an interdisciplinary collaborative review process for the use and care of all central-line catheters (including peripherally inserted central catheters) on this unit, with the primary goal to decrease the incidence of CLABSIs.

The interdisciplinary team included the unit attending physicians, nursing leadership staff, an IP, quality improvement staff, an intravenous therapy clinical nurse specialist, and the unit staff nurses. Through this program, in addition to decreasing the incidence of CLABSIs, the team hoped to increase communications between physicians and nurses regarding the necessity of the central-line catheter and to review the frequency of procedures that require access to the central line. The 8 South Central Line–Associated Bloodstream Infection (CLABSI) Program is an example of a focused intervention that improves patient safety through interdisciplinary bedside rounding, communicating with families, and monitoring the adherence to evidence-based practice standards of care of central lines.

The Problem: Health Care–Associated Bloodstream Infection

Prior to initiating the process improvement, the nurses followed the hospital standards for central-line catheter care; however, at that time, maintaining yearly practice competencies was not required. In addition, changes in practice were occurring that resulted in an increase in central-line catheter days on 8 South. Therefore, as part of a hospitalwide initiative, its HAI rates were monitored more closely. The result was that it had periods of increased infection from April 2007 to January 2008 and again from February 2008 to October 2008 (*see* Case Study Figure 3-1, page 82).

They also noted that physicians and nurses did not communicate regularly about the use of the central-line catheter. A bedside review of CLABSIs convened when two siblings presented with infection. The infectious disease team and nursing staff met with the parent; however, the attending physicians were on bedside rounds in another unit and were not available to meet at that time. In reviewing the case at the bedside, the team identified knowledge deficits in nurses and parents and some procedural concerns related to the use of total parenteral nutrition (TPN) from home. This case became the stimulus for developing a model for bedside review of central-line care with an interdisciplinary team that included the attending physicians.

The nursing leadership staff on 8 South initiated a change in practice at a time when the hospital leadership was organizing teams to evaluate and to change hospitalwide standards of care for central-line catheters. Recognizing that their practice was flawed, leaders immediately began to have mandatory education and observation experiences for all registered nurses. Several staff nurses on 8 South assumed responsibility for the training. The central-line training program consisted of the following: (1) a review of recently revised hospital standards of central-line care, (2) observation of line site dressing change, and (3) mandatory review of a training video that included a post test. The training video provided information on a variety of central-line catheter issues, such as dressing and cap changes, and drawing blood. In addition, the team had weekly meetings with infection control and quality management staff and collaborated with staff from the intravenous team to provide education and a means to certify nurse observers. The nurse manager reviewed the process changes with the attending physicians and asked for nurse and physician involvement in the bedside rounding process.

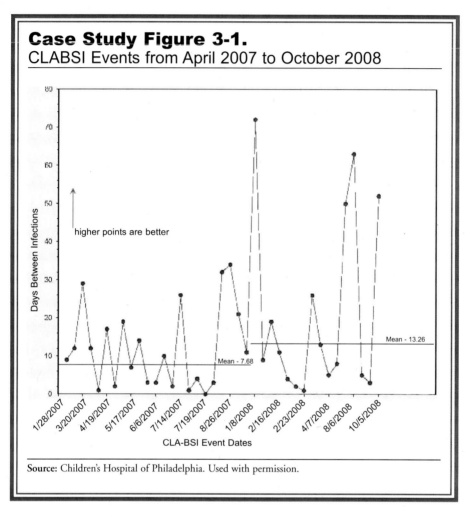

Case Study Figure 3-1.
CLABSI Events from April 2007 to October 2008

Source: Children's Hospital of Philadelphia. Used with permission.

During the time when staff nurses were being educated, a group of nurses developed a brief brochure to educate parents on practice standards and to engage them in the prevention of infection through hand hygiene and securing the central line.

A Culture of Safety
The nurse manager and the clinical nurse specialist on this unit were recruited to join the hospital culture of safety committee and to use their CLABSI Program interventions as tools for modeling a culture of safety. Nursing administrators and

hospital and medical directors supported the endeavor and provided feedback throughout the process. Staff nurses on 8 South maintained a "football field" poster, keeping a running list of the number of infection-free days. They celebrated their successes with support from the attending physicians and other team members. The staff nurses on 8 South now routinely report the status of their central lines; furthermore, they own the responsibility of maintaining central lines that are intact.

Staff buy-in was not a problem. All the nurses on 8 South and throughout the Children's Hospital of Philadelphia strive to provide the best care, and the nursing staff were very receptive to the need for practice changes. Change came easily, because the entire institution was involved in changing practices and implementing facilitywide accountability. The hospital identified the need to have a central-line dressing change cart that is stocked with nonchargeable items and reminders of procedures. It also conducts random audit checks to monitor practices associated with central lines.

Winning the Fight Against Health Care–Associated Infection

The nursing unit at 8 South has received positive feedback from hospital administrators and other units that struggle with CLABSIs. It recently reached 197 days of being free from bloodstream infection; however, on April 21, 2009, it had one patient present with a central line–associated infection. The infected patient had multiple line difficulties (such as a cracked line, no StatLock device, and clotted line) due to having a peripherally inserted central line and additional problems with feeding intolerances. The attending physicians wanted him to have limited line access at home, so they worked on building his feeding tolerance. A team meeting with attending physicians and administrative staff was called to review this challenging case.

Staff Nurses and Health Care–Associated Infection

A body of evidence suggests that staff nurses play significant roles in the spread of infectious diseases in the hospital setting.[3-5] Children's Hospital of Philadelphia presents a model where health care professionals can collaborate in the fight against HAIs, a fight that can be led and won on the front line by registered nurses.

References

1. Klevens R.M., et al.: *Estimating Health Care–Associated Infections and Deaths in U.S. hospitals, 2002.* Public Health Reports, 2007. 122(2): 160–166.
2. Centers for Disease Control and Prevention: Notice to readers: Fourth decennial international conference on nosocomial and healthcare-acquired infections. *MMWR* 49(7):138, 2000.
3. Alonso-Echanove J., et al.: Effect of nurse staffing and antimicrobial-impregnated central venous catheters on the risk for bloodstream infections in intensive care units. *Infect Control Hosp Epidemiol* 24(12):916–925, 2003.
4. Andersen B.M., et al.: Spread of methicillin-resistant *Staphylococcus aureus* in a neonatal intensive unit associated with understaffing, overcrowding, and mixing of patients. *J Hosp Infect* 50(1):18–24, 2002.
5. Stegenga J., Bell E., Matlow A.: The role of nurse understaffing in nosocomial viral gastrointestinal infections on a general pediatrics ward. *Infect Control Hosp Epidemiol* 23(3):133–136, 2002.

Nurses Working with Physicians and Other Licensed Independent Practitioners

Because nurses are not the only clinicians involved in direct patient care, it is essential that they work with physicians and other licensed independent practitioners to prevent and to control infections. One way these clinicians can work together to fight infections is to conduct multidisciplinary unit-based initiatives to prevent specific types of infection. For example, perioperative nurses might team with surgeons and anesthesiologists to develop protocols to reduce the incidence of surgical-site infections (SSIs). Together, the team would review and implement best practices proven to reduce the risk of SSIs and assign responsibility for each step in the process.

Defining Roles and Responsibilities

When multiple disciplines are involved in infection prevention and control, it is important to identify who is responsible for each step of the process. For example, if an organization develops a protocol that requires that surgical patients be given prophylactic antibiotics one hour before surgery, it needs to be clear who should be giving the antibiotic. In some organizations, it may be the nurse. In others, it may be the anesthesiologist.

If it is an organization's policy to screen all patients for methicillin-resistant *Staphylococcus aureus* (MRSA) on admission, the policy should also state who is responsible for doing the nasal swab, who should be informed of the test results, who should initiate contact precautions if necessary, and who should initiate therapy.

Empowering Nurses to Stop Unsafe Practices

Hierarchy can create patient safety risks when nurses are afraid to speak up if a physician is doing something they consider unsafe. When nurses do speak about problems to physicians or leaders, the conversation tends to be indirect and/or deferential. New and inexperienced nurses may be particularly likely to hold back information or concerns for fear of repercussions or due to insecurity about their roles in the hospital or on a team. And senior staff members may resist feedback from someone they view as a subordinate. Although the full effect of hierarchy's negative impact on communication may be difficult to quantify, it can act as a significant barrier to patient safety.[5]

Nurses need to be empowered by leadership to cross hierarchical boundaries when working to stop unsafe practices. If it is the nurse's role to observe staff members and to challenge those who are not adhering to infection prevention and control practices, physicians and staff need to be educated about the proper response to these admonitions. For example, if a nurse sees a physician fail to perform hand hygiene between patients and reminds the physician that he or she missed a hand-hygiene opportunity, a proper response might be, "Thank you for reminding me. I'll go wash up now."

Physician champions who are committed to infection prevention can help break down barriers based on hierarchy. A physician champion who models respect for other team members and openness to their opinions makes a valuable contribution to the team and the overall organizational culture. Champions can ease the way to building collaboration among disciplines and making everyone feel more at ease. For example, a champion may introduce herself using her first name ("Jill Smith") rather than a more formal address ("Dr. Smith") and encourage all other team members, including physicians, to do the same. This helps put everyone on equal footing so they become more comfortable working together.[5]

Although champions and opinion leaders can support patient safety and infection prevention efforts, responsibility for planning and implementing initiatives also rests with leadership. This means establishing teams, giving teams goals, training team members, breaking down hierarchies, and allocating adequate resources.[5]

Nurses Working with Other Patient Care Staff

During the course of a day, nurses work with a multitude of patient care staff, each with the potential to pass infectious agents between patients. Nurses should work closely with other patient care staff, such as physical therapists, radiology technicians, pharmacists, laboratory technicians, respiratory therapists, patient care technicians (PCTs)/certified nursing assistants (CNAs), and nursing students, to use evidence-based principles to prevent and to control infection.

Physical Therapists

Because physical therapists are often in direct contact with their patients, chances for the physical therapist to contract an infectious disease or for cross-contamination between patients are great.[6] However, physical therapists can do a number of things to prevent infection or to decrease the spread of infection. These may include the following[7–10]:

- Practice good hand hygiene.
- Maintain contact precautions; change gowns and gloves between patients.
- Use standard precautions when handling equipment in the patient's room that is likely to have been contaminated.
- When possible, for patients on isolation precautions, dedicate equipment to a single patient.
- If equipment cannot be dedicated to a single patient for patients on isolation precautions, clean it as soon as it is removed from the room.
- For patients on isolation precautions, limit patient movement unless it is essential to treatment.
- Secure urinary catheters properly when moving the patient; maintain free flow for urine.

Nurses can work with physical therapists to ensure that protocols for hand hygiene, contact precautions, patient movement while under contact precautions, and urinary catheter care are being followed. This may include alerting physical therapists to any breeches in infection prevention and control protocols in a nonthreatening and respectful manner. It may also include making sure that catheter bags are being emptied prior to initiation of physical therapy. Nurses can help ensure that protocols are followed by hanging hand-hygiene posters according to organizational protocol; using visual cues, such as signs, to remind other health care workers about contact precautions; and ensuring that gowns and gloves are readily available.

Radiology Technicians

Hospitalized patients frequently need radiology services. The volume of patients moving in and out of the radiology department, the need to reuse expensive equipment, and the need to physically move isolated patients from their rooms to the radiology department (imaging department) create opportunities for the spread of infection. Because they work closely with patients, radiology technicians are also at risk for contracting infectious diseases themselves. Radiology technicians, along with radiologists, can help prevent the spread of infection in the following ways[7-10]:

- Practice good hand hygiene.
- Maintain contact precautions; don gown and gloves before providing radiology services to patients on isolation precautions, and remove them after the patient has been taken from the radiology department.
- Take x-rays in the patient's room whenever possible.
- Clean and disinfect whatever equipment was used as soon as the patient leaves the radiology department or after removing it from the patient's room.
- Secure urinary catheters properly when moving the patient; maintain free flow for urine.

Nurses can work with radiology services to ensure that protocols for hand hygiene, contact precautions, and urinary catheter care are being followed. This may include making sure that catheter bags are being emptied before the patient is sent for imaging studies. If x-rays are being taken in the patient's room, nurses can help ensure that protocols are followed by hanging hand-hygiene posters in areas specified by organizational protocol; using visual cues, such as signs, to remind radiology staff about contact precautions; and ensuring that gowns and gloves are readily available.

Pharmacists

Because many infections are treated by pharmaceutical methods, pharmacists play very important parts in infection prevention and control. Pharmacists are essential in the development of protocols for treating infections and for ensuring that appropriate medications are readily available. Pharmacists can also help educate physicians and patients about the proper use of antibiotics.

Nurses can work with pharmacists by ensuring that patient medication lists are up-to-date. They can also partner with pharmacists by administering medications in a timely manner and documenting patient response to treatment.

Laboratory Technicians

Laboratory technicians come into close contact with blood and bodily fluids on a daily basis, which leaves them not only at risk for cross-contamination between patients but also at risk for contracting infectious diseases themselves. To protect themselves and their patients from the spread of infectious diseases, laboratory technicians can take the following precautions[7–9]:

- Practice good hand hygiene; clean hands before and after obtaining all laboratory samples.
- Maintain contact precautions; don gown and gloves before entering the patient's room, and remove them when leaving.
- Use standard precautions when obtaining blood or bodily fluid samples and when handling blood vials and specimen containers.

Nurses can work with laboratory staff to ensure that protocols for hand hygiene, contact precautions, and standard precautions are being followed. This may include alerting laboratory staff to any noted breeches in infection prevention and control protocols in a nonthreatening and respectful manner. Nurses can help ensure that protocols are followed by hanging hand-hygiene posters according to organizational protocol; using visual cues, such as signs, to remind laboratory technicians about contact precautions; and ensuring that gowns and gloves are readily available.

Respiratory Therapists

Respiratory therapists frequently provide treatments that have the potential to put them in contact with a patient's bodily fluids. Therefore, they run the risk not only of spreading infection from one patient to the next but also of acquiring infections themselves. Respiratory therapists can do several things to protect themselves and their patients against infection. These include the following[7–9,11–13]:

- Practice good hand hygiene.
- Maintain contact precautions; don gown, gloves, and mask before entering the patient's room, and remove them when leaving.
- When possible, dedicate equipment to a single patient.
- If equipment cannot be dedicated to a single patient, clean and disinfect it as soon as it is removed from the room.

- Use an orotracheal tube rather than a nasotracheal tube when possible; secure the tube properly.
- Keep the endotracheal (ET) tube cuff pressure between 20 and 30 cm H2O.
- Suction above and below the ET tube cuff as needed and before ET tube removal.
- Work with physicians to ensure that ET tubes are removed as soon as is clinically feasible.
- For patients who are on ventilators:
  - Keep the head of the bed elevated 30 to 45 degrees, unless contraindicated.
  - Continuously remove subglottic secretions.
  - Change ventilator circuits when visibly soiled or if they are mechanically malfunctioning.

Nurses can work with respiratory therapists and IPs to develop evidence-based protocols for patients who are on ventilators. They may also work together on unit-based projects that may affect both disciplines, such as reducing the incidence of ventilator-associated pneumonia on the unit.

Nurses and respiratory therapists can also work together to ensure that organizationwide protocols for hand hygiene, contact precautions, and standard precautions are being followed. This may include nurses alerting respiratory therapists to any breeches in infection prevention and control protocols in a nonthreatening and respectful manner. Nurses can help ensure that protocols are followed by hanging hand-hygiene posters according to organizational protocol; using visual cues, such as signs, to remind other health care workers about contact precautions; and ensuring that gowns and gloves are readily available.

Patient Care Technicians/Nursing Assistants
PCTs and CNAs are in close contact with patients on a daily basis. Their jobs require that they care for multiple patients on a single day. They are generally the ones who are responsible for helping patients with activities of daily living, including toileting, bathing, and oral care. Their potential for coming in contact with bodily fluids, along with their close proximity to patients, leaves them and their patients vulnerable to the spread of infection. PCTs and CNAs can do a number of things to help prevent and control infection. These include the following[7-11,14]:
- Practice good hand hygiene.

- Maintain contact precautions; don gown and gloves before entering the patient's room, and remove them when leaving. Change gloves and clean hands between patients.
- When possible, dedicate equipment to a single patient.
- If equipment cannot be dedicated to a single patient, clean and disinfect it as soon as it is removed from the room.
- Limit patient movement unless it is essential to treatment.
- Secure urinary catheters properly; maintain free flow to urine.
- Empty catheter bags when they are one-half to two-thirds full.
- Periodically wipe community equipment, such as telephones and computer keyboards, with antibacterial wipes. This is also a responsibility of the environmental services staff.
- Provide frequent oral care.
- Provide catheter care according to organizational protocol.
- Monitor fluid and dietary intake.
- Keep patients' skin clean and dry.

Nurses are responsible for overseeing patient care performed by PCTs and CNAs. Nurses, in collaboration with IPs, should ensure that PCTs and CNAs are adequately trained in the above infection prevention and control practices. They should act as role models for other patient care staff by strictly adhering to hand-hygiene protocols, standard precautions, and contact precautions.

Nursing Students

Nursing students perform many of the same patient care activities as the staff nurses (*see* Chapters 2 and 5). Nurses are responsible for overseeing patient care by students, including oversight of infection prevention and control practices. Nurses should also act as role models for student nurses by strictly adhering to hand-hygiene protocols, standard precautions, and contact precautions.

Nurses Working with Nonclinical Staff

In addition to working with patient care staff, nurses also work with nonclinical staff, who also have the potential to spread infection. Nurses should work closely with nonclinical staff, such as transporters; chaplains; interpreters; engineers, environmental services, and maintenance staff; administrative support staff; and dietitians to assure that each understands his or her role in infection prevention.

What Would You Do?

A transporter enters a patient's room and is preparing to transport the patient to radiology for an x-ray. As the patient is transferred from the bed to a wheelchair, you notice that the patient's catheter bag is almost full. The transporter, who is not wearing gloves, lifts the catheter bag and places it on the patient's lap. She then moves behind the patient and prepares to transport the patient. What would you do?

In this scenario, the full catheter bag and the placement of the catheter bag above the insertion site are both potential risk factors for the patient to develop a UTI. Additionally, the transporter touched the catheter bag without wearing gloves and failed to perform hand hygiene, which can potentially spread infection from the catheter bag to the wheelchair handles, then to other staff members. The nurse might intervene by saying something like, "Here, let me put on some gloves and help you with that while you go wash up." This allows the transporter to see that gloves should be worn and to hear that hand hygiene should be performed when working with patients with catheters. After donning gloves, the nurse should empty the catheter bag and then hang it on the wheelchair below the level of the bladder. As she is hanging the bag, the nurse could say something like, "I'll just hang this down here where it can drain properly, then go wash my hands." This shows the transporter where to hang the catheter bag and reinforces the hand-hygiene message.

Transporters

Transporters frequently come into direct contact with patients as they are assisting them from beds to wheelchairs or gurneys, then to procedures or x-ray tables. Although this is not typically a transporter's role, they may also be asked to assist a patient with toileting, which will increase the transporter's chances of coming into contact with bodily fluids. Transporters can take the following precautions to prevent the spread of infection[6–10]:

- Practice good hand hygiene.
- Maintain contact precautions; don gown and gloves before entering the patient's room, and remove them after handing off the patient at the new location.
- Change gloves and clean hands between patients.

- Secure urinary catheters properly when moving the patient; maintain free flow for urine.

Nurses can work with transporters to ensure that protocols for hand hygiene, standard precautions, and contact precautions are being followed. This may include nurses alerting transporters to any breeches in infection prevention and control protocols in a nonthreatening and respectful manner. It may also include making sure that catheter bags are being emptied prior to transport and teaching transporters how to properly secure urinary catheters. Nurses can help ensure that protocols are followed by hanging hand-hygiene posters according to organizational protocol; using visual cues, such as signs, to remind other health care workers about contact precautions; and ensuring that gowns and gloves are readily available.

Chaplains

Many patients, particularly those who are gravely ill, may feel comforted by speaking to a chaplain. When patients are on isolation precautions and are not able to move freely throughout the facility, the nurse can help by calling the chaplain to visit. Chaplains who are visiting patients in a hospital or other health care facility should be held accountable for appropriate hand-hygiene practices and adherence to standard and contact precautions. Nurses can work with chaplains by alerting them to any breeches in infection prevention and control protocols in a nonthreatening and respectful manner. Nurses can help ensure that protocols are followed by hanging hand-hygiene posters according to organizational protocol; using visual cues, such as signs, to remind other health care workers about contact precautions; and ensuring that gowns and gloves are readily available.

Interpreters

Many patients require the use of an interpreter to fully understand all the elements of their care, treatment, and services. Interpreters are responsible for adhering to appropriate hand-hygiene practices and standard and contact precautions. Nurses can work with interpreters by alerting them to any breeches in infection prevention and control protocols in a nonthreatening and respectful manner. Nurses can help ensure that protocols are followed by hanging hand-hygiene posters according to organizational protocol; using visual cues, such as signs, to remind other health care workers about contact precautions; and ensuring that gowns and gloves are readily available.

Engineers

Dangerous bacteria, fungi, and other infection-causing agents can be spread through an organization's air-handling or water-distribution system. To prevent this, organizations must take a multidisciplinary approach to identifying, evaluating, and addressing the risks involved in utility maintenance. Open communication between nursing and infection control staff and staff in the engineering and maintenance department can help organizations identify risks and address them before they become problems.[2,15]

In addition to maintaining open communication, utility managers should make sure that all utility equipment is properly designed, correctly installed, adequately maintained, and properly functioning. In air-handling and ventilation systems, this means that pressure relationships, air exchange rates, and filtration efficiencies should all be appropriately maintained. This is particularly important in such areas as surgical suites, special procedure and delivery rooms, airborne-infection isolation rooms, sterile supply rooms, and protective isolation rooms where staff care for individuals who have suppressed immune systems.[2,15]

Utility managers should also work with infection preventionists and nurses to educate and train maintenance staff—such as plumbers, painters, and carpenters—who provide routine and emergency maintenance services within an organization. Training should include effective infection control practices, particularly hand hygiene; how to keep equipment and tools clean and sanitary; and guidelines on how and where to store equipment and tools.

Administrative Support Staff

Administrative staff is an important part of the infection control team. In many organizations, they are the ones responsible for making sure that all patients are screened for MRSA by a clinician on admission or before surgical procedures. They may also be responsible for tracking data on staff immunization practices and hospital-acquired infections. In addition, administrative staff can take the following steps to help prevent and control infections[6–9,14]:

- Practice good hand hygiene. Clean hands after using the restroom and before and after handling food.
- Maintain contact precautions; if entering a patient's room, don gown and gloves before entering, and remove them when leaving.

Table 3-2. Tips for Communication Between Dietitians and Other Health Care Professionals During Transitions

Transitioning to the Hospital	Transitioning to Long Term Care	Transitioning to Home Care	Transitioning to Behavioral Health Care
• Pick up the phone and talk to the person who is receiving the patient, preferably a registered dietitian. • Make sure dietary documentation is complete before transferring the patient. • Include information about food allergies and food preferences.	• Make sure a registered dietitian communicates the differences between acute and long term care prior to the physician signing off on the diet order to be used in the new facility. • Send the patient's nutrition assessment and care plan, if available, with the patient each time he or she is transferred. This provides an initial history of the patient's nutritional status, including approaches that have been successful and unsuccessful in treating current nutrition problems. • Include information about food allergies and food preferences.	• If a patient is going home on parenteral nutrition, or tube feeding, communication should be ongoing between the inpatient nutrition support team and the home infusion nutrition support team, including the physicians, nurses, pharmacists, and dietitians. Discuss not only what has been done for the patient in the hospital, but what needs to be continued after discharge. Determine the patient's nutritional goals, and then decide the optimal methods and interventions to achieve them. • Include information about food allergies and food preferences.	• Include registered dietitians in the education of nursing students about nutrition and about the role of the dietitian in discharge planning and hand-off communications. • Include information about food allergies and food preferences. • Physicians and nurses are encouraged to be mindful of the high value of nutrition care and to include registered dietitians in care planning for patients and hand-off communications.

- Periodically wipe community equipment, such as telephones and computer keyboards, with antibacterial wipes.
- Schedule staff training sessions, and notify staff of times and locations.

If administrative staff has reason to enter a patient's room or otherwise have direct contact with a patient, they are responsible for practicing hand hygiene according to organizational protocols and adhering to standard and contact precautions. Nurses can work with administrative staff by alerting them to any breeches in infection prevention and control protocols in a nonthreatening and respectful manner. Nurses can help ensure that protocols are followed by hanging hand-hygiene posters according to organizational protocol; using visual cues, such as signs, to remind other health care workers about contact precautions; and ensuring that gowns and gloves are readily available.

Dietitians

Proper nutrition is vital to infection control, yet information about patients' nutritional dietary needs can frequently become lost during patient transitions or hand-offs, particularly if a patient moves through multiple units or facilities. Table 3-2, page 94, includes tips from registered dietitians that can help ensure good communication between hospital, long term care, home care, and behavioral health care dietitians and other health care professionals.[16]

References

1. Pittet D., Donaldson L.: Challenging the world: Patient safety and health care–associated infection. *Int J Qual Health Care* 18:4–8, Feb. 2006.
2. Joint Commission Resources: Infection control and the environment of care. *The Source* 3:3–5, May 2005.
3. Dawson S.J.: The role of the infection control link nurse. *J Hosp Infect* 54:251–257, Aug. 2003.
4. The Joint Commission: *Comprehensive Accreditation Manual for Hospitals.* Oakbrook Terrace, IL: Joint Commission Resources, 2008.
5. Joint Commission on Accreditation of Healthcare Organizations: *Engaging Physicians in Patient Safety: A Handbook for Leaders.* Oakbrook Terrace, IL: Joint Commission Resources, 2006.
6. McGuckin M.: Evaluation of a patient education model for increasing hand hygiene compliance in an inpatient rehabilitation unit. *Am J Infect Control* 32:235–238, Jun. 2004.
7. Yamamoto L., Marten M.: Listen up MRSA: The bug stops here. *Nursing* 37:51–55, quiz 55–56, Dec. 2007.

8. Cooper E.: VRE: How you can stop the spread of this drug-resistant organism. *RN* 71:27–31, quiz 32, Feb. 2008.
9. Grota P.G.: Perioperative management of multidrug-resistant organisms in health care settings. *AORN J* 86:361–368, quiz 369–372, Sep. 2007.
10. Society of Urologic Nurses and Associates: Clinical practice guidelines: Care of the patient with an indwelling catheter. *Urol Nurs* 26:80–81, Feb. 2006.
11. Pruitt B., Jacobs M.: Best practice interventions: How you can prevent ventilator-associated pneumonia. *Nursing* 36:36–41, Feb. 2006.
12. Kaynar A.M., et al.: Attitudes of respiratory therapists and nurses about measures to prevent ventilator-associated pneumonia: A multicenter, cross-sectional survey study. *Respir Care* 52:1687–1693, Dec. 2007.
13. Tolentino-DelosReyes A.F., Ruppert S.D., Shiao S.Y.: Evidence-based practice: The use of the ventilator bundle to prevent ventilator-associated pneumonia. *Am J Crit Care* 16:20–27, Jan. 2007.
14. Rutala W.A., et al.: Bacterial contamination of keyboards: Efficacy and functional impact of disinfectants. *Infect Control Hosp Epidemiol* 27:372–377, Apr. 2006.
15. Centers for Disease Control and Prevention: *Guidelines for Environmental Infection Control in Health-Care Facilities.* Jun. 6, 2003. http://www.cdc.gov/mmwr/preview/mmwrhtml/rr5210a1.htm (accessed Jul. 31, 2009).
16. The Joint Commission: *Improving Hand-Off Communication.* Oakbrook Terrace, IL: Joint Commission Resources, 2007.

Chapter 4

The Nurse's Role in Educating Patients and Their Families on Safe Infection Prevention and Control Processes

Involving patients and families in decision making and care is an important component of safe and effective care.[1] Therefore, it is critical that patients and families, as well as staff, know that infection prevention and control is everyone's responsibility.[1] Because nurses are frequently patients' primary educators, they have a responsibility to make sure that their patients and their patients' families are educated about infection prevention and control standards within health care settings and at home. This chapter discusses the nurse's role in educating patients about infection prevention and control practices. It includes information about standard precautions and transmission-based precautions. It also discusses education related to specific types of infections and provides educational resources that nurses can use as tools to teach patients about infection prevention and control.

Reporting Concerns

One of the first things that nurses should teach their patients about infection prevention and control is how to report concerns. Reporting systems can be major tools to identify safety issues and to gather information about additional staff education needs.[2]

WHO Guidelines on Adverse Event Reporting

The World Alliance for Patient Safety has commissioned the development of World Health Organization (WHO) guidelines on adverse event reporting and learning systems to help organizations develop or improve reporting systems.[2] The four core principles of the guidelines are as follows[2]:

1. The fundamental role of patient safety reporting systems is to enhance patient safety by learning from failures of the health care system.

2. Reporting must be safe—individuals who report incidents must not suffer any reprisals.
3. Reporting is only of value if it leads to a constructive response. At a minimum, this entails feedback of findings from data analysis. Ideally, it also includes recommendations for changes in processes and systems of health care.
4. Meaningful analysis, learning, and dissemination of lessons learned require expertise and other human and financial resources. The agency that receives reports must be capable of disseminating information, making recommendations for changes, and communicating the development of solutions.

Organizations should keep these principles in mind when developing reporting systems for patients.

Reporting Concerns and Complaints to The Joint Commission

In addition to reporting concerns internally, patient and staff should be made aware that complaints on accredited organizations may also be submitted to The Joint Commission. If a complaint is submitted with a name and contact information, The Joint Commission will notify the person when action is taken in response to the complaint. Complaints may be reported in a number of ways, including the following:

• Online: http://www.jointcommission.org/GeneralPublic/Complaint
• E-mail: complaint@jointcommission.org
• Fax: Office of Quality Monitoring, (630) 792-5636
• Mail: Office of Quality Monitoring, The Joint Commission, One Renaissance Boulevard, Oakbrook Terrace, IL 60181

Complaints should include the name, street address, city, and state of the accredited organization and should be summarized in less than two pages. More information on The Joint Commission complaint process is available by calling (800) 994-6610 (weekdays 8:30 A.M. to 5:30 P.M. central standard time).

Standard Precautions

Standard precautions include a group of infection prevention practices that apply to all patients, regardless of suspected or confirmed infection status, in any setting in which health care is delivered.[3] These include hand hygiene; use of gloves, gown, mask, eye protection, or face shield, depending on the anticipated exposure; and safe injection practices.[3]

Hand Hygiene

Germs that can cause serious illnesses are easily transmitted when an infected person touches surfaces that other people have touched.[4] Nurses come into contact with numerous types of infectious organisms. Patients should feel empowered to ask nurses if they have cleaned their hands before they provide any type of treatment or service that will require contact with the patients.[5] "It is our responsibility as professionals to provide education about hand hygiene," says Barbara M. Soule, R.N., M.P.A., C.I.C., practice leader, Infection Prevention and Control, Joint Commission Resources. "Patients and families have a right to ask caregivers if they've washed their hands and to expect a respectful response."

Maryanne McGuckin, Dr.Sc.Ed., M.T. (A.S.C.P.), president, McGuckin Methods International, Inc., and senior scholar, Department of Health Policy, Jefferson Medical College, Philadelphia, says that getting patients to remind health care workers to clean their hands is the single-most-important thing that organizations can do to improve hand-hygiene practices. "Our research over the last 10 years has documented that 85% of patients said they would ask their health care worker to wash or sanitize their hands before treating them, but in reality, only 70% actually did," she says. McGuckin also notes that four out of five consumers said they would have no problem asking their health care workers to wash or sanitize their hands if invited to do so.[6]

Nurses should teach their patients to clean their own hands using soap and warm water. If their hands do not look dirty, they can be cleaned with alcohol-based hand sanitizers.[5] Hand hygiene should be performed before touching or eating food and after using the bathroom.[5] Patients should also be taught to perform hand hygiene at the following times[4,7]:

- After contact with blood or bodily fluids
- After changing a baby's diaper
- After handling pets, their toys, leashes, or waste
- After touching something that could be contaminated (for example, a trash can, cleaning cloth, or soil)
- After spending time in a public place
- When hands are visibly dirty
- After coughing, sneezing, or blowing their noses
- Before and after touching cuts, burns, or infected wounds
- Before, during, and after interacting with someone who is sick

Proper Hand-Hygiene Techniques

Many people, including some nurses, do not know the proper techniques for performing hand hygiene. Nurses should be educated about hand-hygiene techniques so they can teach their patients the following methods for hand washing and using alcohol-based gels[4,7]:

Hand Washing

1. Wet your hands with warm water, and apply liquid, bar,* or powder soap.
2. Rub hands together vigorously to make a lather, and scrub all surfaces. Do not forget to scrub between the fingers and around the nails.
3. Continue for 20 seconds (about the time it takes to sing "Happy Birthday" twice).
4. Rinse hands well under running water.
5. Dry hands using a paper towel or air dryer.
6. If possible, use the paper towel to turn off the faucet.

Using Alcohol-Based Gels

1. Make sure the solution covers all the surfaces of the hands.
2. Rub hands together vigorously. Do not forget the area between the fingers and around the nails.
3. Rub the solution in until it has evaporated and hands are dry.

Tools for Educating Patients and Families About Hand Hygiene

The following tools can help nurses educate patients and families about hand hygiene:

- **"Hand Hygiene Saves Lives" Video.** This video, developed by the Centers for Disease Control and Prevention (CDC), is available in English and Spanish. It teaches two key points to hospital patients and visitors to help prevent infections: that it is important to practice hand hygiene while in the hospital and that it is appropriate to ask or to remind healthcare providers to practice hand hygiene as well. Available at http://www.cdc.gov/handhygiene/.
- **Hand Hygiene Posters** (*see* Figures 4-1, page 101, and 4-2, page 102). Available at http://www.cdc.gov/print.do?url=http://www.cdc.gov/handhygiene/Patient_Admission_Video.html.
- **Hand Hygiene Brochures** (*see* Figure 4-3, page 103). Available at http://www.cdc.gov/print.do?url=http://www.cdc.gov/handhygiene/Patient_Admission_Video.html.

For more information about standard precautions, *see* Chapter 1.

---

* When bar soap is used, soap racks that facilitate drainage and small bars of soap should be used. Please see the CDC Hand Hygiene Guidelines for more information.

Figure 4-1. Hand Hygiene Poster (English Version)

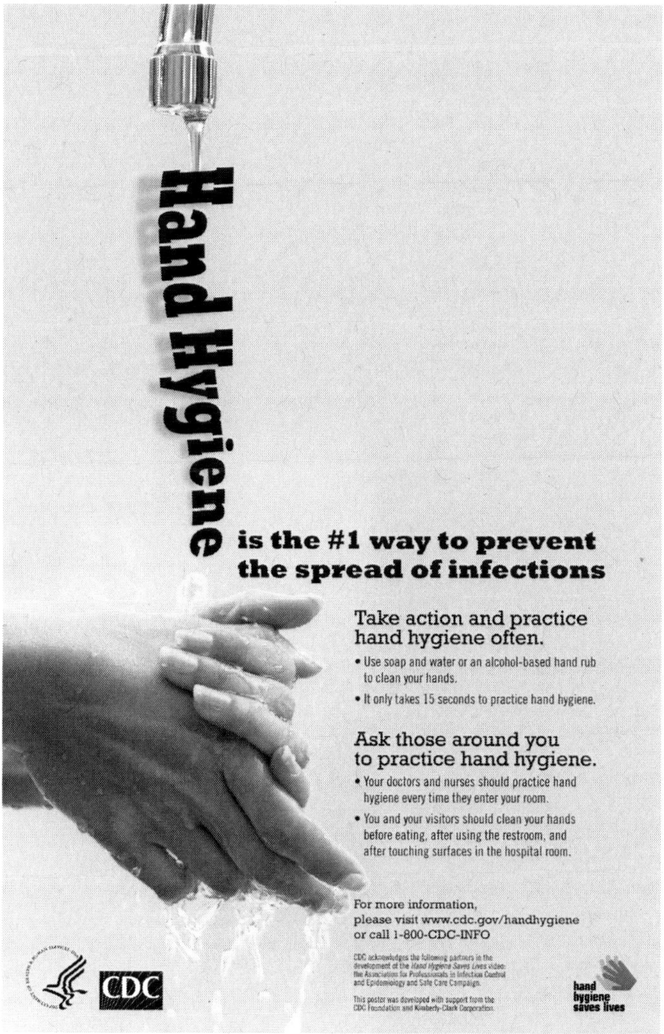

The posters in Figures 4-1 and 4-2 are designed to educate patients about hand-hygiene practices.

Source: Centers for Disease Prevention and Control. Available at http://www.cdc.gov/handhygiene (accessed Jun. 9, 2009).

Figure 4-2. Hand Hygiene Poster (Spanish Version)

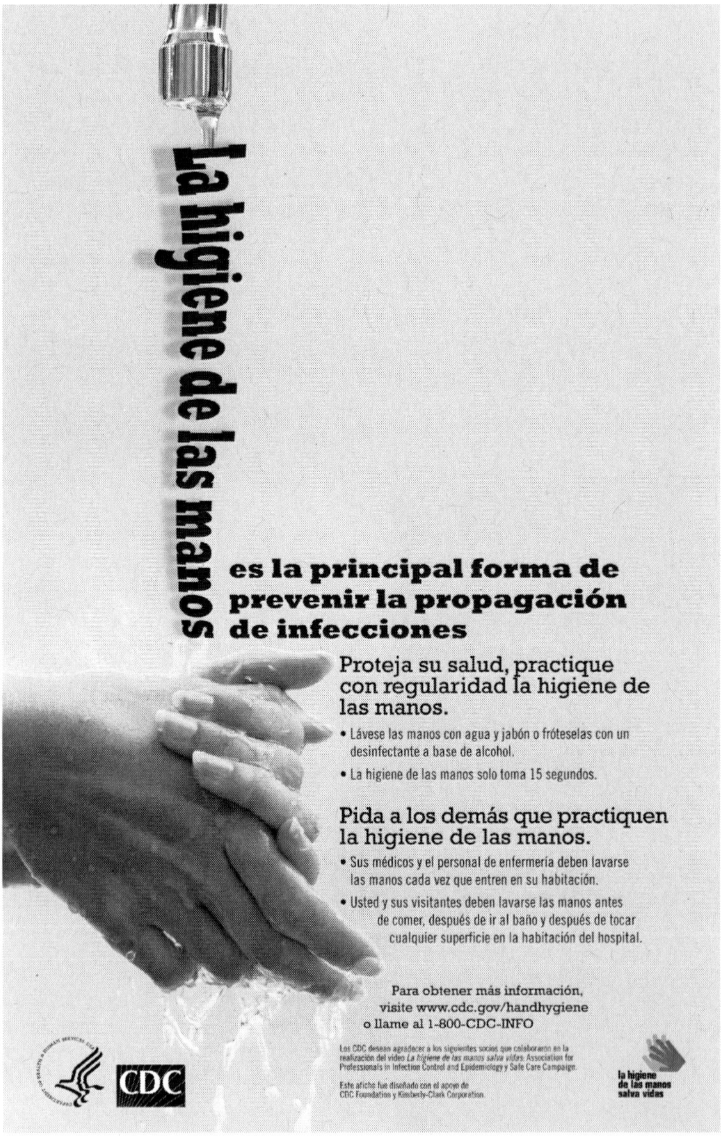

Source: Centers for Disease Prevention and Control. Available at http://www.cdc.gov/handhygiene (accessed Jun. 9, 2009).

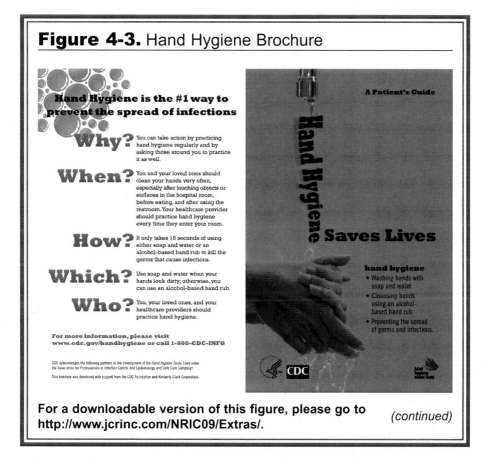

Figure 4-3. Hand Hygiene Brochure

For a downloadable version of this figure, please go to http://www.jcrinc.com/NRIC09/Extras/. *(continued)*

Respiratory Hygiene/Cough Etiquette

Many diseases are spread through airborne pathogens. When a patient sneezes or coughs, the germs can travel three feet or more.[5] Patients should be taught to cover their mouths and noses to prevent the spread of droplet and airborne infections. "The purpose of respiratory hygiene is to prevent organisms from being transmitted through talking, sneezing, or coughing," says Soule. "Patients should be taught to always try to cover their mouth and nose with a handkerchief or tissue when sneezing or coughing. If they don't have a handkerchief or tissue available, they should cough into their sleeve. They should also wash their hands frequently. If they are ill, patients may need to wear a mask when moving about the organization."

Figure 4-3. Hand Hygiene Brochure, *continued*

Why?

To prevent hospital infections.
- In the United States, hospital patients get nearly 2 million infections each year. That's about 1 infection per 20 patients!
- Infections you get in the hospital can be life-threatening and hard to treat.
- All patients are at risk for hospital infections.
- You can take action by asking both your healthcare providers and visitors to wash their hands.

Remember: Hand hygiene saves lives.

To make a difference in your own health.
- Hand hygiene is one of the most important ways to prevent the spread of infections, including the common cold, flu, and even hard-to-treat infections, such as methicillin-resistant *Staphylococcus aureus*, or MRSA.

When?

You should practice hand hygiene:
- Before preparing or eating food.
- Before touching your eyes, nose, or mouth.
- Before and after changing wound dressings or bandages.
- After using the restroom.
- After blowing your nose, coughing, or sneezing.
- After touching hospital surfaces such as bed rails, bedside tables, doorknobs, remote controls, or the phone.

Healthcare providers should practice hand hygiene:
- Every time they enter your room.*
- Before putting on gloves. Wearing gloves alone is not enough to prevent the spread of infection.
- After removing gloves.

Remember: Ask your doctors and nurses to clean their hands before they examine you.

* If you already have an infection, your healthcare providers may take special measures (isolation precautions) to prevent the spread of your infection to others. They might enter your room wearing protective equipment (e.g., gloves, gown, mask). You do not need to ask them to clean their hands because they should have done so before they put on gloves.

How?

With soap and water:
1. Wet your hands with warm water. Use liquid soap if possible. Apply a nickel- or quarter-sized amount of soap to your hands.
2. Rub your hands together until soap forms a lather and then rub all over the top of your hands, in between your fingers and the area around and under the fingernails.
3. Continue rubbing your hands for 15 seconds. Need a timer? Imagine singing the "Happy Birthday" song twice.
4. Rinse your hands well under running water.
5. Dry your hands using a paper towel if possible. Then use your paper towel to turn off the faucet and to open the door if needed.

Remember: It only takes 15 seconds to protect yourself and others.

With an alcohol-based hand rub:
1. Follow directions on the bottle for how much of the product to use.
2. Rub hands together and then rub product all over the top of your hands, in between your fingers and the area around and under the fingernails.
3. Continue rubbing until your hands are dry. If enough rub was used to kill germs, it should take at least 15 seconds of rubbing before your hands feel dry. You should not rinse your hands with water or dry them with a towel.

Which?

Use soap and water:
- When your hands look dirty.
- After you use the bathroom.
- Before you eat or prepare food.

Use an alcohol-based hand rub:
- When your hands do not look dirty.
- If soap and water are not available.

Alcohol-based hand rubs
- Products that kill germs on the hands.
- Should contain 60% to 95% ethanol or isopropanol (types of alcohol).
- Are fast-acting and convenient.

Who?

You can make a difference in your own health:
- Healthcare providers know they should practice hand hygiene, but they sometimes forget. Most welcome your friendly reminder.
- Ask healthcare providers to practice hand hygiene in a polite way — tell them that you know how easy it is for people to get infections in the hospital and that you don't want it to happen to you.

Remember: Take control of your health; practice hand hygiene.

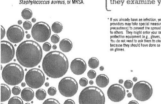
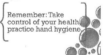

This brochure can be provided to patients on admission to a facility.

Source: Centers for Disease Prevention and Control. Available at http://www.cdc.gov/handhygiene/PDF/CDC_HandHygiene_Brochure.pdf (accessed Dec. 2, 2009).

Transmission-Based Precautions

Health care–associated infections (HAIs) are a serious safety challenge for health care organizations. One way some organizations address HAIs is through the use of standard precautions, as well as transmission-based precautions, that are employed to reduce the risk of disease transmission and HAIs based on the specific method of organism transmission.[8]

Transmission-based precautions should be implemented when the route(s) of transmission is (are) not completely interrupted using standard precautions alone.[3]

According to the CDC, three categories of transmission-based precautions exist: contact precautions, droplet precautions, and airborne precautions.[3] Transmission-based precautions are always used in addition to standard precautions.[3]

Contact Precautions

Contact precautions are applied for patients who are infected or colonized with multidrug-resistant organisms (MDROS).[3] Contact precautions also apply when a patient has excessive wound drainage, fecal incontinence, or other discharges from the body that would suggest an increased potential for extensive environmental contamination and risk of transmission.[3]

People who are sick should be taught to be careful when coming in contact with other people. "Contact precautions are sometimes necessary to stop the transmission of organisms through direct or indirect contact with the patient," says Sylvia Garcia-Houchins, R.N., M.B.A., C.I.C., consultant, Joint Commission Resources. "Precautions include frequent hand hygiene, and sometimes gowns, gloves, and masks. Patients need to be told that they have contracted an organism that has been known to be transmitted through contact so they know why it is important for health care workers and visitors to take appropriate precautions. They also need to be told to remind visitors and staff to wear protective equipment."

Nurses should wear clean gloves when they perform such tasks as taking throat cultures, taking blood, touching wounds or bodily fluids, or examining a patient's mouth or private parts. Patients should not be afraid to ask nurses to put on gloves.[5]

Droplet Precautions

The purpose of droplet precautions is to prevent transmission of pathogens spread through close contact with respiratory secretions.[3] Droplet precautions are indicated for patients who have been diagnosed with *B. pertussis,* influenza virus, adenovirus, rhinovirus, *N. meningitides,* and group A streptococcus (for the first 24 hours of antimicrobial therapy).[3] A single-patient room is preferred for patients on droplet precautions, if available. If a single-patient room is not available, other patient placement options, such as cohorting or keeping the patient with an existing roommate, may be considered.[3] Patients on droplet precautions who must be transported outside the room should wear surgical cone masks, if tolerated, and follow respiratory hygiene/cough etiquette as described on page 103.[3]

Airborne Precautions

Airborne precautions are used to prevent transmission of infectious agents that remain infectious over long distances when suspended in the air. These may include measles, chicken pox, Mycobacterium tuberculosis, and SARS-CoV.[3] Patients who require airborne precautions should be placed in an airborne infection isolation room (AIIR). In health care settings where airborne precautions cannot be implemented due to limited resources (for example, a physician's office), the patient should be masked and placed in a private room with the door closed.[3] Health care providers should be provided with N95 or higher level respirators, or masks if respirators are not available, until the patient is either transferred to a facility with an AIIR or returned home.[3] Health care personnel caring for patients on airborne precautions should don masks or respirators, depending on the disease-specific recommendations, prior to room entry.[3] Whenever possible, nonimmune health care workers should not care for patients with vaccine-preventable airborne diseases (for example, measles, chicken pox, and smallpox).[3]

Educating Patients About Transmission-Based Precautions

Education better enables patients and family to comply with isolation protocols and also gives them a sense of what will occur and why. For example, nurses should educate their patients about why they need to wear surgical masks if they must be transported to other areas in the facility for tests and why keeping visitors to a minimum is important. Patients educated about why care providers must wear protective gowns and gloves with contact isolation can participate in ensuring their safety by insisting that a staff member don appropriate attire before entering the room to provide care.[8]

Nurses should be aware of and sensitive to the experience of infectious patients in isolation. Documented patient responses to isolation include feelings of neglect, abandonment, punishment, and imprisonment.[8] Depression and anxiety, which are experienced to some degree by many isolated patients, constitute patient safety concerns for individuals at risk for suicide and restraint. Disorientation due to the lack of stimuli can be of particular concern with elderly isolated patients at risk for falls in hospitals and long term care facilities.[8]

Real or perceived communication barriers can impact patients and staff and, therefore, patient safety. Patients may be uncertain that their requests for help using call lights have been noted, especially when long waits are experienced. The need to put on protective clothing certainly elongates response time a bit, and nurses, if unable to observe patients directly, experience more challenges in anticipating patient needs. Leaders can address the effects on staff of caring for isolated patients through proper staffing and staff education. Patient education, as described earlier, can also help reduce some of the psychological effects of isolation that put patients at risk for harm.[8]

Tools to Educate Patients About Transmission-Based Precautions
The following tools can help nurses educate their patients about transmission-based precautions:

- **Contact Precautions Patient Information Sheet.** Developed by the University of California San Francisco (*see* Figure 4-4, page 108).
- **Hospital Patient and Family Contact Precautions Information Sheet.** Developed by the Winnipeg Regional Health Authority. Available at http://www.wrha.mb.ca/healthinfo/a-z/aro/infosheet.php.
- **Droplet Precautions Patient Information Sheet.** Developed by the University of California San Francisco (*see* Figure 4-5, page 109).
- **Droplet Isolation: Infection Control Brochure.** Developed by the U.S. Department of Veteran's Affairs. Available at http://www.centraltexas.va.gov/patients/Patient-Education-Handouts/Droplet-Precautions.pdf.
- **Airborne Precautions Patient Information Sheet.** Developed by the University of California San Francisco (*see* Figure 4-6, page 110).
- **Patient/Family Education Routine Airborne Precautions Information Sheet.** Developed by Children's Hospitals and Clinics of Minnesota. Available at http://www.childrensmn.org/Manuals/PFS/TestProc/058292.pdf.

Patient Hygiene

Because germs carried on the skin or in the mouth can cause infections, patient hygiene also plays a key role in reducing infections. Patient and family education related to good hygiene practices should include the following:

- **Oral hygiene.** Regular oral care can help reduce plaque, which can cause infection. Education related to oral hygiene should include proper tooth brushing, flossing, denture care, and nutrition and hydration. Dry lips that are cracked can be a portal for infection, so oral hygiene should include the use of nonpetroleum lip lubricants.[9]
- **Bathing.** Bathing is one of the first activities of daily living that becomes difficult for the elderly.[6] Bathing can be facilitated by the use of bath aids, such as grab

Figure 4-4. Contact Precautions Information Sheet

UC_{SF} Medical Center 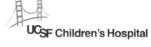 UC_{SF} Children's Hospital

Contact Precautions Patient Information

Everyone has germs. Most of them are harmless, some are helpful. A few germs, however, can make you sick. At UCSF Medical Center and Children's Hospital, our goal is to protect our patients, their families and visitors from germs that might make them sick. In the hospital, precautions are used as a way of stopping the spread of germs from one person to another. This page should help answer questions you/your family may have.

? What are "Contact Precautions"?
You have been placed on "Contact Precautions" because you have (or may have) germs in or on your body that can be harmful to other people. These germs are spread when people touch you or your environment, or when you touch others.

? What will the hospital staff do?
• Clean their hands frequently
• Put a GREEN "STOP" sign on your door to let staff entering your room know what to do.
• Wear gloves when entering your room and gowns when they may contact you or your environment.

? What can I do to help?
• **Clean your hands often.**
• Be sure visitors entering your room have read the sign on your door.
• Limit your visitors to a few family members or close friends.

? What should my visitors do?
• **Clean their hands upon entering and exiting your room.**
• Avoid contact with your dressings, urine bag, tubes, or bed sheets, etc.
• Go to the nurse's station if they have any questions.
Because your visitors don't go into the rooms of other patients,
they don't need to wear gowns & gloves while visiting you!

? How do I clean my hands correctly?

Use soap and water:
• Wet hands with warm water
• Dispense one measure of soap into palm.
• Work up lather by rubbing hands together for 15 seconds, covering all surfaces of the hands and fingers.
• Rinse hands thoroughly
• Dry hands with paper towel.
• Use a towel to turn off faucet.
• Discard towel in the trash container.

Use Alcohol Gel:
• Dispense one measure of gel into palm of one dry hand
• Rub hands together covering all surfaces of hands and fingers until dry, about 15 – 20 seconds.
• If you have *C. difficile*, soap and water hand cleaning is recommended.

It is okay to remind our staff to clean their hands!
Department of Hospital Epidemiology and Infection Prevention and Control 415-353-4343

This patient information sheet can help nurses educate their patients about contact precautions.

Source: Used with permission of the Department of Hospital Epidemiology and Infection Control, Amy D. Nichols, R.N., M.B.A., C.I.C., director, University of California at San Francisco Medical Center and Children's Hospital, San Francisco, CA.

Figure 4-5. Droplet Precautions Information Sheet

UC_{SF} Medical Center

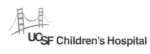 UC_{SF} Children's Hospital

Droplet Precautions Patient Information

Everyone has germs. Most of them are harmless, some are helpful. A few germs, however, can make you sick. At UCSF Medical Center and Children's Hospital, our goal is to protect our patients, their families and visitors from germs that might make them sick. In the hospital, precautions are used as a way of stopping the spread of germs from one person to another. This page should help answer questions you/your family may have.

? What are "Droplet Precautions"?
You have been placed on "Droplet Precautions" because you have (or may have) germs in your lungs or throat can be harmful to other people. These germs are spread to other people by the droplets sprayed from your mouth or nose when you speak, sneeze or cough, and can also be picked up when people touch the surfaces around you.

? What will the hospital staff do?
- Clean their hands frequently
- Put a YELLOW "STOP" sign on your door to let staff entering your room know what to do.
- Wear a mask and eye protection when within 3 feet of you ("arm's reach").
- Place masks outside your door for use by hospital staff and visitors.

? What can I do to help?
- **Clean your hands often, especially after coughing and sneezing.**
- Be sure visitors entering your room have read the sign on your door.
- Leave your room only when medically necessary and <u>wear a mask whenever you do</u>.
- Limit your visitors to a few family members or close friends. **Siblings of pediatric patients on Droplet precautions are discouraged from visiting the nursing unit.**

? What should my visitors do?
- **Clean their hands upon entering and exiting your room.**
- Put on a mask & eye protection before entering the room and keep it on while inside (recommended).

? How do I clean my hands correctly?

Use soap and water:
- Wet hands with warm water
- Dispense one measure of soap into palm.
- Work up lather by rubbing hands together for 15 seconds, covering all surfaces of the hands and fingers.
- Rinse hands thoroughly
- Dry hands with paper towel.
- Use a towel to turn off faucet.
- Discard towel in the trash container.

Use Alcohol Gel:
- Dispense one measure of gel into palm of one dry hand
- Rub hands together covering all surfaces of hands and fingers until dry, about 15 – 20 seconds.

It is okay to remind our staff to clean their hands!
Department of Hospital Epidemiology and Infection Prevention and Control 415-353-4343

This patient information sheet can help nurses educate their patients about droplet precautions.

Source: Used with permission of the Department of Hospital Epidemiology and Infection Control, Amy D. Nichols, R.N., M.B.A., C.I.C., director, University of California at San Francisco Medical Center and Children's Hospital, San Francisco, CA.

Figure 4-6. Airborne Precautions Information Sheet

UC_{SF} Medical Center   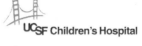 UC_{SF} Children's Hospital

Airborne Precautions Patient Information

Everyone has germs. Most of them are harmless, some are helpful. A few germs, however, can make you sick. At UCSF Medical Center and Children's Hospital, our goal is to protect our patients, their families and visitors from germs that might make them sick. In the hospital, precautions are used as a way of stopping the spread of germs from one person to another. This page should help answer questions you/your family may have.

? What are "Airborne Precautions"?
You have been placed on "Airborne Isolation" because you have (or may have) germs in your lungs or throat that can be harmful to other people. These germs are spread by tiny droplets from your mouth or nose that stay suspended in the air and can be breathed in by other people.

? What will the hospital staff do?
- Clean their hands frequently
- Put a **PINK** "STOP" sign on your door to let staff entering your room know what to do.
- Keep your door closed.

? What can I do to help?
- **Clean your hands often, especially after coughing and sneezing.**
- Keep your door closed at all times.
- Be sure visitors entering your room have read the sign on your door.
- Leave your room only when medically necessary and <u>wear a mask whenever you do</u>.
- Limit your visitors to a few family members or close friends immune to your communicable illness.

? What should my visitors do?
- **Clean their hands upon entering and exiting your room.**
- Be certain they are immune to your communicable illness (vaccinated or already had the disease).
- Go to the nurse's station if they have any questions.

? How do I clean my hands correctly?

Use soap and water:
- Wet hands with warm water
- Dispense one measure of soap into palm.
- Work up lather by rubbing hands together for 15 seconds, covering all surfaces of the hands and fingers.
- Rinse hands thoroughly
- Dry hands with paper towel.
- Use a towel to turn off faucet.
- Discard towel in the trash container.

Use Alcohol Gel:
- Dispense one measure of gel into palm of one dry hand
- Rub hands together covering all surfaces of hands and fingers until dry, about 15 – 20 seconds.

It is okay to remind our staff to clean their hands!
Department of Hospital Epidemiology and Infection Prevention and Control 415-353-4343

This patient information sheet can help nurses educate their patients about droplet precautions.

Source: Used with permission of the Department of Hospital Epidemiology and Infection Control, Amy D. Nichols, R.N., M.B.A., C.I.C., director, University of California at San Francisco Medical Center and Children's Hospital, San Francisco, CA.

bars, shower seats, tub stools, bath chairs, handheld shower sprays, and nonskid mats. Patients should be assessed for bathing disabilities and provided with adequate tools to assist them.[10,11]

- **Incontinence management.** Patients who are incontinent are at increased risk for skin breakdown and subsequent infection. Education should include keeping the skin clean and dry and assessing for skin breakdown.
- **Wound care.** To keep wounds free from infection, patients and caregivers should be taught good hand-hygiene practices, methods for cleaning and dressing the wound, signs and symptoms of wound infection (pain, redness, swelling, increased drainage, foul odor, fever), and who to contact if any problems develop.[12]

Supplies/Equipment

Patients with infectious diseases or surgical wounds need to be educated about the possible transmission of infection through equipment, supplies, or common surfaces. Equipment or surfaces that are frequently touched by others (for example, door knobs, telephones, television remote controls) should be cleaned and disinfected according to the manufacturer's instructions.[13] Equipment can be cleaned using soap and water, diluted bleach, or premixed disinfectants that can be purchased from a store.[13]

Patients with wounds should be instructed to keep dressing supplies in their original packages until it is time to change their dressings.[13,14]

For people with MDROs, laundry should be washed and dried on the hottest suitable temperature, according to label instructions. People with MDROs should not share washcloths, towels, or other personal items.[13]

Influenza

On average, 5% to 20% of the population gets influenza every year in the United States; more than 200,000 people are hospitalized from influenza complications; and about 36,000 people die from flu.[15] The elderly, young children, and people with certain health conditions are at high risk for serious influenza complications.[15]

Many people do not realize that influenza is a respiratory virus and mistakenly use the word "flu" when they are having gastrointestinal (GI) symptoms. It is important that nurses make the distinction between influenza and gastroenteritis ("stomach flu") when educating patients about influenza.

The best way to prevent the flu is by getting an annual flu vaccination. Anyone who wants to reduce his or her chances of getting influenza can be vaccinated. However, it is recommended that people who are at high risk of having serious influenza complications or people who live with or care for those at high risk for serious complications be vaccinated each year. Those who should be vaccinated include the following[16]:

- Children ages 6 months to 19 years
- Pregnant women
- People ages 50 and older
- People of any age with certain chronic medical conditions, such as heart disease, lung disease, or a disease that may weaken the immune system
- People who live in nursing homes and other long term care facilities
- People who live with or care for those at high risk for complications from influenza, including the following:
  – Health care workers
  – Household contacts of persons at high risk for complications from influenza
  – Household contacts and out of home caregivers of children less than 6 months old

People who should not be vaccinated without consulting a physician include the following[16]:

- People who have a severe allergy to chicken eggs
- People who have had a severe reaction to an influenza vaccination
- People who developed Guillain-Barré syndrome within six weeks of getting an influenza vaccine
- Children less than 6 months old
- People who have a moderate-to-severe illness with a fever (they should wait until they recover and no longer have a fever to get vaccinated)

In addition to being given information about the influenza vaccine, patient education should include information about the appropriate use of antibiotics (*see* Figure 4-7, page 113). It should also include the following influenza prevention methods[17]:

- Avoid close contact with people who have respiratory symptoms (for example, coughing and sneezing).
- Stay at home when you are sick.
- Wash your hands frequently.
- Avoid touching your eyes, nose, or mouth.

Figure 4-7. Get Smart: Know When Antibiotics Work

What Everyone Should Know and Do
Snort. Sniffle. Sneeze. No Antibiotics Please!

Are you aware that colds, flu, most sore throats, and bronchitis are caused by viruses? Did you know that antibiotics do not help fight viruses? It's true. Plus, taking antibiotics when you have a virus may do more harm than good. Taking antibiotics when they are not needed increases your risk of getting an infection later that resists antibiotic treatment.

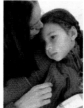

If You Have a Cold or Flu, Antibiotics Won't Work For You!

Antibiotics kill bacteria, not viruses, such as:

Colds or flu
Most coughs and bronchitis
Sore throats not caused by strep
Runny noses

Taking antibiotics for viral infections, such as a cold, cough, flu, or most bronchitis, will not:
Cure the infections
Keep other individuals from catching the illness
Help you feel better

"As a doctor and a mom, I know how sick you or your child can feel with a virus, but antibiotics just won't help. Talk with your doctor or nurse to find out what can help."

Dr. Cyndy Whitney, CDC's Respiratory Diseases Branch Chief.

What Can I Do to Protect Myself or My Child?

When you use antibiotics appropriately, you do the best for your health, your family's health, and the health of those around you. "We want Americans to keep their families and communities healthy by getting smart about the proper use of antibiotics," said Lauri Hicks, D.O., medical director of CDC's "Get Smart" campaign.

This handout can help educate health care workers about the appropriate use of antibiotics.

(continued)

Tools for Educating Patients and Families About Influenza Prevention

The following tools can help nurses educate patients and families about preventing influenza:

- **Poster Discouraging Visits from People with Respiratory Symptoms.** Developed by Bethesda Health (*see* Figure 4-8, page 115).
- **"Take 3" Steps to Fight the Flu Poster.** Developed by the CDC (*see* Figure 4-9, page 116).
- **Health Care Provider "Vaccinated Against Flu. I Care About You" Stickers.** Developed by the CDC. Available at http://www.cdc.gov/flu/professionals/flugallery/2008-09/healthcare_provider_stickers.htm.

Figure 4-7. Get Smart: Know When Antibiotics Work, *continued*

What to Do

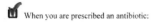 Talk with your health care provider about antibiotic resistance.

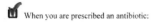 When you are prescribed an antibiotic:

1. Take it exactly as the doctor tells you. Complete the prescribed course even if you are feeling better. If treatment stops too soon, some bacteria may survive and reinfect you.
2. This goes for children, too. Make sure your children take all medication as prescribed, even if they feel better.
3. Throw away any leftover medication once you have completed your prescription.

What Not to Do

 Do not take an antibiotic for a viral infection, such as a cold, cough, or flu.

 Do not demand antibiotics when a doctor says they are not needed. They will not help treat your infection.

 When you are prescribed an antibiotic:

1. Do not skip doses.
2. Do not save any antibiotics for the next time you get sick
3. Do not take antibiotics prescribed for someone else. The antibiotic may not be appropriate for your illness. Taking the wrong medicine may delay correct treatment and allow bacteria to multiply.

Dangers of Antibiotic Resistance

Antibiotic resistance has been called one of the world's most pressing public health problems. It can cause significant danger and suffering for people who have common infections that once were easily treatable with antibiotics. When antibiotics fail to work, the consequences include longer-lasting illnesses, more doctor visits or extended hospital stays, and the need for more expensive and toxic medications. Some resistant infections can cause death.

Sick individuals are not the only people who can suffer the consequences. Families and entire communities feel the impact when disease-causing germs become resistant to antibiotics. These antibiotic-resistant bacteria can quickly spread to family members, schoolmates and coworkers, threatening the community with a new strain of infectious disease that is more difficult to cure and more expensive to treat.

Source: Centers for Disease Prevention and Control. Available at http://www.cdc.gov/getsmart/antibiotic-use/know-and-do.html (accessed Dec. 2, 2009).

Figure 4-8. Influenza Prevention Poster

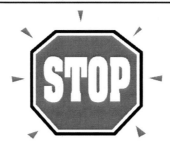

TO PROTECT OUR RESIDENTS, WE ASK THAT YOU NOT VISIT IF YOU HAVE ANY FLU-LIKE SYMPTOMS
SUCH AS FEVER, COUGH, RUNNY NOSE.

THANK YOU FOR YOUR COOPERATION

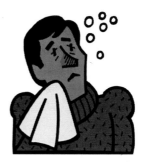

This poster will alert visitors to stay at home when sick to avoid the spread of influenza.

Source: Bethesda Medical Center. Used with permission.

Figure 4-9. "Take 3" Steps to Fight the Flu

CDC Says: "Take 3" Steps to Fight the Flu

Flu is a serious contagious disease.
Each year in the United States, on average:
- More than 200,000 people are hospitalized from flu complications.
- 20,000 of those hospitalized are children younger than 5 years old.
- 36,000 people die from flu.

The Centers for Disease Control and Prevention (CDC) urges you to take the following steps to protect yourself and others from influenza (the flu):

 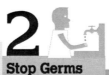 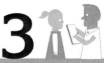

1 Vaccinate
- Take time to get a flu vaccine.
- CDC recommends a yearly flu vaccine as the first and most important step in protecting against this serious disease.
- While there are many different flu viruses, the flu vaccine protects against the three main flu strains that research indicates will cause the most illness during the flu season.
- The vaccine can protect you from getting sick from these three viruses or it can make your illness milder if you get a different flu virus.
- Getting a vaccine is very important for people at high risk for serious flu complications, including young children, pregnant women, people with chronic health conditions like asthma, diabetes or heart or lung disease, and people 65 years of age and older.
- People who live with or care for those at high risk should also get a flu vaccine to protect their high-risk contact.

2 Stop Germs
- Take everyday preventive actions.
- Cover your nose and mouth with a tissue when you cough or sneeze. Throw the tissue in the trash after you use it.
- Wash your hands often with soap and water, especially after you cough or sneeze. Alcohol-based hand cleaners are also effective.
- Try to avoid close contact with sick people.
- If you get the flu, CDC recommends that you stay home from work or school and limit contact with others to keep from infecting them.
- Avoid touching your eyes, nose or mouth. Germs spread this way.

3 Antiviral Drugs
- Take flu antiviral drugs if your doctor recommends them.
- If you do get the flu, antiviral drugs are an important treatment option. (They are not a substitute for vaccination.)
- Antiviral drugs are prescription medicines (pills, liquid or an inhaler) that fight against the flu by keeping flu viruses from reproducing in your body.
- Antiviral drugs can make your illness milder and make you feel better faster. They may also prevent serious flu complications. This could be especially important for people at high risk.
- For treatment, antiviral drugs work best if started soon after getting sick (within 2 days of symptoms).
- Flu-like symptoms include fever (usually high), headache, extreme tiredness, dry cough, sore throat, runny or stuffy nose and muscle aches.

 For more information about flu, visit **www.cdc.gov/flu**

This poster can help to educate patients and families about the prevention and treatment of influenza.

Source: Centers for Disease Prevention and Control. Available at http://www.cdc.gov/flu/freeresources/ (accessed Jun. 9, 2009).

What Would You Do?

A man is recovering from a minor surgical procedure. His son, daughter-in-law, and grandson come to visit him. His daughter-in-law is suffering from what appears to be a bad cold and, although hospital policies prohibit children under the age of 10 from visiting patients in this ward, the 3-year-old grandson still came up.

You notice that the woman is sneezing and coughing into her hands. You also notice that the child keeps moving from his mother's lap to the patient's lap in the hospital bed. In addition, you observe that the woman is changing the television stations on the remote control to find something the child can watch. What would you do?

In this scenario, infection may be spread from the mother to the child to the patient, as the child moves from the mother's lap to the patient's bed. It may also be spread from the mother's hands to the remote control to the patient. The nurse should take this opportunity to educate the patient and the family members about preventing the spread of infection. The nurse might say something like, "I notice that you seem to have a bad cold, and I am concerned that you may pass it on to your father-in-law, which could complicate his recovery. Because germs are often spread by contact, anything you touch can potentially spread germs from you to your father-in-law. I know that you came here out of concern, and I appreciate that you [the patient] might want to see your family, but it is best if you [the daughter-in-law] wait to visit until you are over your cold." The nurse might go on to say, "Perhaps you were unaware, but we also have a policy that does not allow children under the age of 10 on this ward, so I'll have to ask that you leave your child at home when you return."

This statement allows that the daughter-in-law has good intentions but clearly states how her illness can be spread to her father-in-law, impeding his recovery. It also allows that she may not have known about the organization's policy about children under the age of 10 but gives her no wiggle room if she brings the child a second time.

Multidrug-Resistant Organisms

As noted in Chapter 2, the incidence of MDROs, such as methicillin-resistant *Staphylococcus aureus* (MRSA), vancomycin-resistant enterococci (VRE), and *Clostridium difficile (C. diff),* has steadily increased over the past four decades.[18–20] MDROs cause infections that are difficult and costly to treat and that result in increased morbidity and mortality.[18] Nurses should teach their patients about the importance of staying at home when they have illnesses that could be potentially infectious.

Patients and families can do many things to decrease the likelihood of infection from MDROs. This chapter discusses how nurses can involve patients and families in the prevention of MDROs.

Methicillin-Resistant Staphylococcus Aureus

More than 7% of the U.S. population has MRSA, but many are unaware.[21] MRSA is a resistant strain of the common bacterium *Staphylococcus aureus,* commonly known as *staph.* Some people may have an infection triggered by MRSA or they can carry the bacteria on their skin or in their nasal passages without having any symptoms. Even if no symptoms are present, carriers of MRSA can infect others if the germ makes contact with open wounds. MRSA currently accounts for 40% to 60% of *S. aureus* infections.[21] It is most frequently found in patients with immune systems that have been weakened by age, disease, or invasive medical procedures.

Most patients are infected through hand contact, particularly from nurses or other health care workers. However, recent literature has reported the occurrence of community-associated MRSA in postpartum women and neonates.[5] Outbreaks have also been reported in healthy, full-term newborns presenting with MRSA infection after discharge from normal newborn nurseries.[22] "In 1998, the first official report of MRSA in people with no known risk factors was released following the deaths of four children," says Jeremias Murillo, M.D., hospital epidemiologist, Newark Beth Israel Medical Center, Newark, New Jersey. "In the past, MRSA had always been associated with health care exposure. These were the first known cases of community-acquired MRSA. We now have more patients coming into the hospital already infected with MRSA. Some are chronic patients, but we're seeing an increasing number who have had no recent exposure to health care."

Preventing the Spread of MRSA in the Community and Health Care Facility

Patients and families can do many things to help prevent the spread of MRSA. These include the following[23–25]:

- Wash hands frequently; use alcohol-based hand gel if soap and water are not available.
- Clean minor cuts with soap and water; apply an antibiotic ointment and a bandage.
- Bathe or shower daily.
- Do not share towels, washcloths, razors, or other personal items.
- Wash clothes and soiled linens in hot water.
- Disinfect nondisposable items that may have come in contact with the infected area with a household disinfectant.
- Cover the mouth and nose with a tissue when coughing or sneezing.
- Do not participate in contact sports until all sores have healed.
- Do not go to a public gym, sauna, hot tub, or pool until all sores have healed.
- Tell all health care providers that you have had MRSA in the past.

Tools for Educating Patients and Families About MRSA

A number of tools are available that can help nurses educate patients and families about MRSA. These include the following:

- **Living with MRSA.** A patient education brochure developed by GroupHealth Cooperative, the Tacoma/Pierce County Health Department, and the Washington State Department of Health. Available at http://www.ihi.org/NR/ rdonlyres/C70733CE-8C97-4BFE-880B-13322BD29B72/0/ LivingwithMRSAHandbook.pdf.
- **Patient Information Sheet.** Developed by St. Clare's Health System. Available in English and Spanish (*see* Figures 4-10, page 120, and 4-11, page 121).
- **MRSA Patient Fact Sheet.** Developed by the CDC (see Figure 4-12, page 122).
- **Learning About MRSA: A Guide for Patients. Developed by the Minnesota Department of Health.** Available at http://www.health.state.mn.us/divs/ idepc/diseases/mrsa/book.pdf.
- **"Protect Yourself from MRSA" Poster.** Developed by the Michigan Department of Community Health and the Michigan Antibiotic Resistance Coalition (*see* Figure 4-13 on page 123).
- **MRSA Brochure.** Developed by Bethesda Health (*see* Figure 4-14, page 124).

Figure 4-10. MRSA Patient Information Sheet (English Version)

PATIENT INFORMATION

Information supplied by www.cdc.org

MRSA *(Methicillin Resistant Staphylococcus Aureus)*

You have just been told that you or your family member has a MRSA infection. What does this mean? How will this be treated? What precautions to I need to take? Please take a moment to review this information. Please do not hesitate to ask your physician, nurse or our Infection Control nurses if you have any further questions.

What is MRSA?

Staphylococcus (Staph) aureus is a germ that lives on your skin. When you are healthy, your body's immune system keeps these germs in check and keeps them from making you sick. When your resistance is low because you are taking antibiotics for another infection or you are in the hospital, the *Staphylococcus aureus* can get into open wounds, your blood, your urine or your sputum and cause an infection. Sometimes germs become resistant to certain antibiotics which mean those particular antibiotics will not stop the infection. When *Staph aureus* shows resistance to an antibiotic called Methicillin, it is called MRSA.

How is it found?

Your physician has ordered either a test of your blood, wound, urine or sputum which has confirmed that you have the MRSA germ present. This may either be an active infection which means you are showing signs of an infection (fever, pneumonia, high white blood cell counts, or drainage from a wound) or you are colonized with the germ which means it is in your body but you have no clinical signs of an infection.

Why do I need to be isolated?

When you are a patient in a hospital, your body has a lower immune system. The staff at the hospital needs to prevent the spread of germs between patients. Since MRSA is an organism that is resistant to many antibiotics, special care needs to be utilized to prevent spreading this particular germ to other patients. You will be placed in a private room if it is available (at no extra cost to you). A sign will be placed outside your door alerting staff and visitors to use special precautions. Staff will wear gloves and gown and maybe use a mask when caring for you. As the patient, you should also wash your hands frequently. You can still walk around the unit as long as the site of your infection is contained/covered.

Can my family and friends still visit me?

You can still have visitors, but ask visitors to speak with your nurse about any special precautions they may need to take. Visitors will be asked to wash their hands when they are leaving your room. Friends and family who are ill themselves should not come to visit.

What precautions do I need to take when I go home?

When you go home, no special precautions need to be utilized. You must use good hand washing techniques. Any special precautions will be reviewed with you by your physician and your nurse before you go home.

What if I come back to the hospital?

It is important to let your physician and nurse know that you have had MRSA. You may be placed in isolation when you arrive and lab tests done to see if the MRSA is still present on your system. If it is not, then you can be removed from isolation.

Pease do not hesitate to discuss your questions or concerns with your physicians or nurses. You may also ask your nurse to call the Epidemiology Department if you have any specific questions or concerns 973-625-6597 or 6598 or 973-983-5549. Thank you.

† CATHOLIC HEALTH
INITIATIVES®

Saint Clare's Health System

This one-page information sheet, available in English and Spanish, can help health care providers educate patients about MRSA.

Source: St. Clare's Health System. http://www.ihi.org/NR/rdonlyres/EA3EF598-3062-4206-9CB0-772BE4204B89/0/MRSAenglish.pdf. Used with permission.

For a downloadable version of this figure, please go to http://www.jcrinc.com/NRIC09/Extras/.

Figure 4-11. MRSA Patient Information Sheet (Spanish Version)

MRSA (Methicillin Resistant Staphylococcus Aureus)

Acaban de informarle que usted o un familiar tiene una infección de MRSA. ¿Qué significa esto? ¿Cómo se tratará? ¿Qué precauciones necesito tomar? Por favor, tómese un momento para repasar esta información y no vacile en hablar con su médico, enfermera, o nuestras enfermeras de Control de infección si tiene más preguntas.

¿Qué es MRSA?

Staphylococcus (Staph) es una bacteria que vive en la piel. Cuando está sano, el sistema inmunitario del cuerpo controla estas bacterias para que no lo hagan enfermar. Cuando su resistencia es baja porque está tomando antibióticos para otra infección o está en el hospital, el Staphylococcus aureus puede introducirse en lesiones abiertas, en la sangre, orina o esputo, y producir una infección. A veces las bacterias se vuelven resistentes a algunos antibióticos, o sea que esos antibióticos particulares no detendrán la infección. Cuando Staph aureus muestra resistencia a un antibiótico llamado Methicillin, se llama MRSA.

¿Cómo se descubre?

Su médico ha ordenado un análisis de sangre, lesión, orina o esputo que ha confirmado que tiene presente la bacteria de MRSA. Esto puede ser una infección activa, o sea que usted manifiesta síntomas de infección (fiebre, neumonía, números elevados de glóbulos blancos en la sangre, o drenaje de una herida), o que está colonizado con la bacteria, es decir que la tiene en el cuerpo, pero no manifiesta ningún síntoma clínico de infección.

¿Por qué necesito estar aislado?

Cuando usted está internado en el hospital, el cuerpo tiene un sistema inmunitario más bajo y el personal del hospital debe impedir que se contagien los pacientes. Como MRSA es un organismo resistente a muchos antibióticos, se necesita un cuidado especial para impedir que esta bacteria en particular contagie a otros pacientes. Se le pondrá en una habitación privada si la hay disponible (sin cobrarle más) y se colocará un letrero afuera de su puerta alertando a personal y a las visitas para que tomen las precauciones necesarias. El personal llevará guantes y bata y quizás use una mascarilla al hacerle tratamiento. Como paciente, usted debe lavarse las manos con frecuencia; aun así, puede caminar por la unidad siempre y cuando esté contenido o tapado el lugar de la infección.

Aun así, ¿pueden visitarme familiares y amigos?

Sí puede tener visitas, pero pídales que hablen con la enfermera sobre las precauciones que necesiten tomar. Se les pedirá a las visitas que se laven las manos al salir de su habitación. Amistades y familiares que se encuentran ellos mismos enfermos no deben venir de visita.

¿Qué precauciones necesito tomar cuando vuelva a casa?

Cuando vuelva a su casa, no tendrá que tomar precauciones especiales; debe lavarse bien las manos. El médico y la enfermera repasarán con usted toda precaución que fuera necesaria antes de que se vaya.

¿Qué pasa si vuelvo al hospital?

Es importante informar a su médico y enfermera que ha tenido MRSA. Es posible que lo pongan en aislamiento cuando llegue y le hagan pruebas de laboratorio para ver si todavía está presente MRSA en su organismo. Si no es así, podrán sacarlo de aislamiento.

Por favor no vacile en hablar con sus médicos y enfermeras sobre sus preguntas e inquietudes. También puede pedirle a la enfermera que llame al Departamento de epidemiología si tiene preguntas o inquietudes específicas, al 973-625-6597 o 6598 o 973-983-5549. Gracias.

Este documento ha sido traducido del inglés al español. Los dialectos regionales y locales pueden diferir. Si necesita ayuda para entender esta planilla, por favor comuníquelo a un representante del hospital.

† CATHOLIC HEALTH INITIATIVES®

Saint Clare's Health System

This one-page information sheet, available in English and Spanish, can help health care providers educate patients about MRSA.

Source: St. Clare's Health System. http://www.ihi.org/NR/rdonlyres/A39F2277-4395-4ECB-BE2F-6377FAC7CE70/0/MRSAspanish.pdf. Used with permission.

For a downloadable version of this figure, please go to http://www.jcrinc.com/NRIC09/Extras/.

Figure 4-12. MRSA Patient Fact Sheet

Have you been diagnosed with a *Staphylococcus aureus* or MRSA infection?
Below are answers to some common questions...

What is *Staphylococcus aureus* or Staph?

Staph is a type of bacteria. It may cause skin infections that look like pimples or boils. Skin infections caused by Staph may be red, swollen, painful, or have pus or other drainage. Some Staph (known as Methicillin-Resistant *Staphylococcus aureus* or MRSA) are resistant to certain antibiotics, making it harder to treat. The information on this page applies to both Staph and MRSA.

Who gets Staph infections?

Anyone can get a Staph infection. People are more likely to get a Staph infection if they have:
- Skin-to-skin contact with someone who has a Staph infection
- Contact with items and surfaces that have Staph on them
- Openings in their skin such as cuts or scrapes
- Crowded living conditions
- Poor hygiene

How serious are Staph infections?

Most Staph skin infections are minor and may be easily treated. Staph also may cause more serious infections, such as infections of the bloodstream, surgical sites, or pneumonia. Sometimes, a Staph infection that starts as a skin infection may worsen. It is important to contact your doctor if your infection does not get better.

How are Staph infections treated?

Treatment for a Staph skin infection may include taking an antibiotic or having a doctor drain the infection. If you are given an antibiotic, be sure to take all of the doses, even if the infection is getting better, unless your doctor tells you to stop taking it. Do not share antibiotics with other people or save them to use later.

How do I keep Staph infections from spreading?

- Wash your hands often or use an alcohol-based hand sanitizer
- Keep your cuts and scrapes clean and cover them with bandages
- Do not touch other people's cuts or bandages
- Do not share personal items like towels or razors

If you have any questions about your condition, please ask your doctor.
For more information, please visit: http://www.cdc.gov/ncidod/dhqp/ar_mrsa.html.

This one-page patient information form developed by the CDC includes information about how to stop the spread of MRSA.

Source: Centers for Disease Prevention and Control. Available at http://www.cdc.gov/mrsa (accessed Jun. 9, 2009).

Figure 4-13. Protect Yourself from MRSA and Other Infections

Protect Yourself From MRSA and Other Infections
Methicillin-resistant *Staphylococcus aureus*

Personal Hygiene
- Wash hands before preparing food, before eating, before and after touching wounds or bandages, after using the bathroom, after coughing/sneezing/blowing your nose, or whenever hands are visibly soiled.
- Shower daily – always after working out – dry off with your own clean towel and put on clean clothes.
- Do not share personal items, like towels, bar soap, wash cloths, razors, clothing or jars of ointment – even among family members.
- Use clothing or a towel as a barrier between skin and shared surfaces, like exercise equipment.

Hand Hygiene
- Wash with soap and water and scrub for at least 15 seconds. Dry with a clean cloth or paper towel, or forced warm air.
- An alcohol-based hand sanitizer containing 61% or more alcohol, like Purell®, may also be used to clean hands when soap and water aren't available and hands aren't visibly dirty.

Respiratory Hygiene
- Cover your mouth and nose with a tissue or your shirt sleeve when sneezing or coughing.

Wound Care
- Keep wounds clean, dry and covered with a fresh bandage.
- Avoid touching other people's wounds or soiled bandages.
- Throw away soiled bandages.
- Watch for signs of infection. If a cut or scrape becomes red, swollen, painful, warm to the touch, or starts draining pus, see a healthcare provider immediately.
- If wound drainage can't be fully contained under a bandage, avoid close contact with others (work, school, sports activities) to prevent the spread of MRSA.

Antibiotics
- Use antibiotics only as directed by a healthcare provider.
- Don't take antibiotics for viral infections, like colds and flu.
- Take antibiotics exactly as prescribed.
- Don't save antibiotics for later or share them with others.

Laundry
- Wash clothes, towels and sheets in water (at hottest suitable temperature) with laundry detergent. Add bleach, if desired (check label instructions). Dry in a dryer at hottest suitable temperature – do not "line dry."

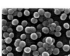

Cleaning
- Clean and disinfect high-touch or soiled surfaces (for example, door knobs and phones frequently, and shared sports equipment between uses) according to item label cleaning instructions. Types of cleaning/disinfecting products include soap and water, diluted bleach, Lysol®, and Original Pine-Sol®. Follow label instructions for appropriate dilutions and contact times to be sure that surfaces are cleaned properly.

for more information visit these Web sites

MDCH **MARR**
Protecting our antibiotic lifeline.

www.michigan.gov/mdch · **www.reducemisuse.org**

This poster was made possible with support from the Michigan Department of Community Health and the Michigan Antibiotic Resistance Reduction Coalition.
© 2006 MDCH and MARR Coalition

This poster can help educate patients about protecting themselves from MRSA.

Source: Michigan Department of Community Health and the Michigan Antibiotic Resistance Coalition. Used with permission.

Figure 4-14. Methicillin-Resistant *Staphylococcus aureus* (MRSA) Brochure

Questions?

_____
_____
_____
_____
_____
_____
_____
_____
_____
_____
_____
_____
_____
_____
_____
_____
_____

Please ask your nurse
Or doctor if you have any
Questions.

Bethesda Health Group
Form # 8870-428-Y-B-D-PA 5/08

**Methicillin
Resistant
Staphylococcous
Aureus
(MRSA)**

The Bethesda Staff
hopes that you find the
following information
helpful during your
stay. Please ask your
nurse or doctor if you
have any questions,
Thank You.

This brochure can be provided to patients and families as a tool to educate them about MRSA.

(continued)

Vancomycin-Resistant Enterococci

Vancomycin is often used to treat infections caused by enterococci, bacteria that are normally present in the human intestines and in the female genital tract.[26] Enterococci can cause infections of the urinary tract, surgical site, or bloodstream.[27] In some cases, enterococci can become resistant to vancomycin.[26]

VRE is often passed from person to person via nurses or other caregivers who have not performed appropriate hand hygiene between patients. VRE can get onto a caregiver's hands after they have contact with other people with VRE or after contact with contaminated surfaces. VRE can also be spread directly to people after they touch surfaces that are contaminated with VRE.[26]

Figure 4-14. Methicillin-Resistant *Staphylococcus aureus* (MRSA) Brochure, *continued*

What is MRSA?

Staphylococcus aureus, often referred to simply as "staph," is a type of bacteria commonly found on the skin and in the nose of healthy people.

- Occasionally, the staph bacteria can get into the body and cause an infection. This infection can be minor (such as pimples, boils or other skin conditions) or serious (such as blood infection or pneumonia).

- Methicillin is an antibiotic commonly used to treat staph infections. Although methicillin is very effective in treating most staph infections, some staph bacteria have developed resistance to methicillin and can no longer be killed by this antibiotic. These resistant bacteria are called Methicillin Resistant Staphylococcus Aureus (MRSA).

What is the difference between colonization and infection?

- Colonization means that MRSA is present on or in the body without causing illness.

- Infection means that MRSA is making the person sick.

Is MRSA Treatable?

- Yes. Although MRSA is resistant to many antibiotics and often difficult to treat, a few antibiotics can still successfully treat MRSA infections.

- Patients who are only colonized with MRSA usually do not need treatment.

Can MRSA spread?

- Yes. MRSA can spread among other patients who are often very sick with weak immune systems who may not be able to fight off infections. MRSA is almost always spread by physical contact, and not through the air.

- Healthcare facilities usually take special steps to prevent the spread of MRSA from patient to patient. One of these steps is to separate, or isolate a patient with MRSA from other patients.

What happens when a patient with MRSA or history of MRSA is isolated?

Procedures vary from one facility to another.

1. Health care workers wear gloves (and sometimes gowns) before entering the patient's room, remove their gloves (and gowns) and wash hands before leaving the room.

2. Visitors do not need to wear gloves or gowns continuously. Visitors may be asked to wear gloves (and sometimes gowns) if they are helping to take care of the patient and are likely to come in contact with the patient's skin, blood, urine, wound, or other body substances.

3. Visitors should always wash their hands before leaving the patient's room to make sure they don't take MRSA out of the room with them.

Is it safe to be in the same room with a person with MRSA?

- Healthy people are at very little risk of getting infected with MRSA. As long as family members or other visitors are healthy, it is okay for them to be in the same room with a person with MRSA. Casual contact, such as touching or hugging also is okay. However, be sure to wash your hands before you leave the residents room to reduce the likelihood that you will become colonized.

- Persons who are very ill or who have weak immune systems should avoid handling the body substances of a person with MRSA and should limit their physical contact to no more than casual touching. They should also wash their hands after physical contact with a person with MRSA.

Can my family get MRSA by being around a person with MRSA?

Healthy people, including children, are at very little risk of getting infected with MRSA.

If you are infected or colonized with MRSA, you should take the following precautions to prevent spreading MRSA to your family and others:

- Follow good hygiene practices, as described earlier.

- Tell any nurses or doctors who treat you that you have MRSA.

Source: Bethesda Health. Used with permission.

Preventing the Spread of VRE

Patients and families can do many things to help prevent the spread of VRE. These include the following[26,28,29]:

- Ask friends and family to wash their hands before and after visiting; in the hospital, visitors may be asked to wear gowns and gloves.
- Wash hands thoroughly after using the bathroom and before preparing food. Clean hands after contact with persons who have VRE.
- Do not share dishes and utensils.
- Frequently clean areas of the home, such as the bathroom, that may become contaminated with VRE.
- Wear gloves if a possibility exists of coming in contact with body fluids that may contain VRE, such as stool or bandages from infected wounds. Wash hands after removing gloves.

- Put all disposable wastes (for example, dressings and bandages) into plastic bags before throwing them in the garbage.
- Wash clothes separately if soiled with body fluids; use detergent with bleach.
- Tell all health care providers that you have VRE.

Tools for Educating Patients and Families About VRE

A number of tools are available that can help nurses educate patients and families about VRE. These include the following:
- **Information for the Public About VRE. Developed by the CDC.** Available at http://www.cdc.gov/ncidod/dhqp/ar_VRE_publicFAQ.html.
- **Patient/Family Information Sheet.** Developed by Greenwich Hospital. Available at http://www.greenhosp.org/pe_pdf/genmed_vre.pdf.
- **Patient Education for VRE Brochure.** Developed by The Christ Hospital (*see* Figure 4-15, page 127).

Clostridium Difficile

Until recently, *C. diff* was never at the top of anyone's list of reportable diseases. Rates of severe disease and death were historically 3% or less,[30] which may explain why *C. difficile*–associated disease (CDAD) was considered to be a fairly low priority. The diseases associated with *C. diff* infection include the following[30]:
- Diarrhea (in which *C. diff* is the cause of 15% to 25% of all cases of antibiotic-associated diarrhea)
- Colitis (in which *C. diff* is responsible for 50% to 70% of antibiotic-related colitis cases)
- Toxic megacolon
- Colonic perforation
- Sepsis

To cause disease, *C. diff* must be present in the GI tract. Indeed, it may remain in a healthy person's system without causing disease until the normal flora in the large intestine is changed, usually through antibiotic use, whether for treatment of infection or as prophylaxis before surgery. Several factors increase a patient's risk of developing CDAD when *C. diff* is present in his or her system[30]:
- Use of antibiotics, including cephalosporins, penicillins, clindamycin, and fluoroquinolones
- GI surgery/procedures, including manipulation of the GI tract, GI or bowel surgery, or use of a nasogastric tube or tube feedings

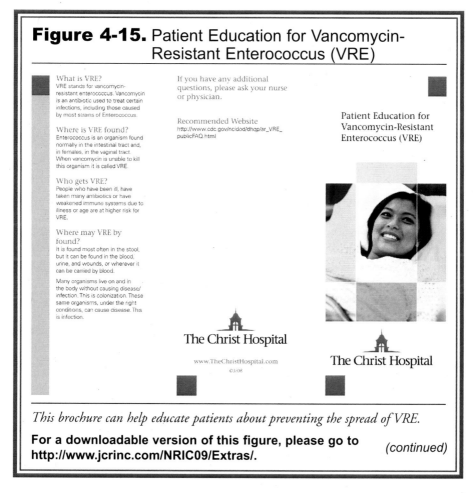

Figure 4-15. Patient Education for Vancomycin-Resistant Enterococcus (VRE)

This brochure can help educate patients about preventing the spread of VRE.

For a downloadable version of this figure, please go to http://www.jcrinc.com/NRIC09/Extras/. *(continued)*

- Extended length of stay in a health care setting(s)
- Advanced age (>60 years)
- Presence of a serious underlying illness, including cancer, renal disease, acquired immune deficiency syndrome (AIDS), diabetes, and other diseases that can compromise a patient's immune system

Patient Education

One of the most important preventive strategies an organization can use is to give patients the information they need to become involved in their own care. However, patients who receive antibiotics as outpatients may not report symptoms immediately,

Figure 4-15. Patient Education for Vancomycin-Resistant Enterococcus (VRE), *continued*

How can VRE be treated?
Some VRE can be treated with antibiotics if that patient is infected. Often, if the patient is colonized, he or she is not treated with drugs.

Patients sometimes get rid of VRE on their own as their bodies get healthier and they are taken off antibiotics. With most patients this takes a few months.

How can VRE be spread?
It can be spread to other people by contact between persons. To prevent this from happening:

1. Contact isolation is used when VRE colonization or infection is identified. An isolation sign will be placed on your door to alert staff and visitors of the special precautions. Healthcare workers and visitors should wear gloves and gowns when they are caring for you; and should also wash hands before and after having contact with you.

2. VRE is a very hardy organism. It can survive on hard surfaces for five to seven days and on hands for hours. It is easy to kill with good handwashing and the proper use of disinfectants. It does not travel through the air; so facial masks are not needed.

3. Your room surfaces and equipment will be kept clean with disinfectants.

What visitors should know?
Healthy visitors and family members should wear gowns and gloves when they visit you in the hospital. All visitors and family members should wash hands thoroughly upon entering and before leaving room and avoid visiting other patient areas during the same visit. Clothing can be taken home and laundered in the usual way.

How long will I have VRE?
No one knows for sure. Some people can carry VRE in their intestinal tract indefinitely. When you enter a healthcare facility or clinic, let the staff know that you have had VRE. A swab may be obtained from your stool or rectal area to determine if you still have VRE.

What do I need to do at home?
Your nurse will review good hygiene practices with you before you go home. You need to do those until your doctor or nurse tells you that you no longer have VRE.

Home Care
Wash your hand for at least 10-15 seconds after close contact with a VRE patient or with any items the patient has touched, and before making and food and before eating.

- Wear rubber gloves if you must handle stool or urine. Wash your hands after taking off the gloves.

- Do not share dishes and utensils.

- Wash your hands before eating.

- If you have no dishwasher, wash the dishes with dish soap and hot water; rinse with hot water and allow to air dry.

Cleaning your house
You can use a solution of bleach and water to clean contaminated surfaces. Mix one part bleach to 10 parts water. You should make up a new batch each day. If you'd rather, you can use any commercial disinfectant cleaner.

VRE is easy to kill on surfaces as long as it is in contact with disinfectant cleaner for enough time. If you wet a surface well with cleaner and let it air dry that should be enough contact time to kill the germ.

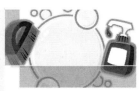

If possible, the patient should have his or her own bathroom. If not, clean the toilet and sink at least daily. Be especially careful to clean after bowel movements.

Laundry
Wash the patient's clothing separately if they are soiled with body fluids; use detergent with bleach.

Clothes not soiled with body fluids can be washed with the family's clothing.

Waste management
Put all disposable wastes like dressings and bandages into plastic bags. Tie the bags securely. They can be thrown out with the regular garbage.

Doctor's Appointments
When you go to the doctor's offices or to hospital appointments, you should tell the doctors and nurses that you have VRE so they can take steps to avoid spreading it to others.

Source: The Christ Hospital. http://www.thechristhospital.com/upload/docs/Departments/InfectionControl/Patient%20Education%20for%20VRE%20brochure%2028030.pdf. Used with permission.

because they may not associate new abdominal problems with antibiotic use, believing they simply have "the flu" or some other ailment that will resolve itself.

Those who contract CDAD and remain untreated and/or continue taking the high-risk antibiotic are more likely to experience more serious outcomes, such as pseudomembranous, fulminant colitis, or toxic megacolon.[30] Registered nurses can assist licensed independent practitioners to monitor patients' antibiotic use. For example, if protocol dictates that antibiotics be discontinued 48 hours after a patient has a negative culture, the nurse can alert the licensed independent practitioner if the antibiotic has not been discontinued within that time frame.

Nurses can also help educate patients and families about the possibility of complications related to antibiotic use, including CDAD. Researchers in Pennsylvania found that many patients who were discharged from the hospital developed symptoms after release.[30] This illustrates the need for strong patient education about *C. diff;* patients must know what to look for so they will consult physicians if they develop symptoms rather than ignoring possible danger signals.

NPSG.07.03.01 also requires that as of January 1, 2010, organizations educate patients, and their families as needed, who are infected and colonized with an MDRO about HAI strategies.

Tools for Educating Patients and Families About *Clostridium Difficile*

Nurses can use the following resources to help educate patients and families about *C. diff:*
- *Clostridium difficile* **Fact Sheet for patients.** Developed by the CDC (*see* Figure 4-16, page 130).
- *Clostridium difficile* **Brochure.** Developed by Bethesda Health (*see* Figure 4-17, page 132).

Surgical Site Infections

It is estimated that the cost of surgical-site infections (SSIs) is about $1.6 billion annually.[31] Although a wealth of knowledge about how to prevent SSIs is available, that information is often not shared with patients.[31,32] What patients need to know about SSIs can be broken down into what should be done before, during, and after surgery. However, because patients may not be at their best immediately after surgery, they should be educated before their surgical procedures, should receive written instructions at discharge, and should be instructed throughout their care.

Before Surgery

Nurses should teach their patients to take the following steps before surgery to help prevent SSIs[32–35]:
- Avoid elective procedures if you have an existing infection.
- Ask questions so that you fully understand your treatment plan and expected outcomes.
- Stop smoking for as long as possible before surgery. Smoking increases the risk for SSIs.

Figure 4-16. *Clostridium difficile* Fact Sheet

What is *Clostridium difficile (C. diff)*?

Clostridium difficile [klo-STRID-ee-um dif-uh-SEEL] is a bacterium that causes diarrhea and more serious intestinal conditions, such as colitis.

What are *C. diff* diseases?

They are diseases that result from *C. diff* infections, such as colitis, more serious intestinal conditions, sepsis, and rarely death.

What are the symptoms of *C. diff* disease?

Symptoms include:
- Watery diarrhea (at least three bowel movements per day for two or more days)
- Fever
- Loss of appetite
- Nausea
- Abdominal pain/tenderness

How is *C. diff* disease treated?

C. diff is generally treated for 10 days with antibiotics prescribed by your healthcare provider. The drugs are effective and appear to have few side effects.

How do people get *C. diff* disease?

People in good health usually do not get *C. diff* disease. People who have other illnesses or conditions requiring prolonged use of antibiotics and the elderly are at greater risk of acquiring this disease. The bacteria are found in feces. People can become infected if they touch items or surfaces that are contaminated with feces and then touch their mouths or mucous membranes. Health care workers can spread the bacteria to other patients or contaminate surfaces through hand contact.

What should I do to prevent spreading *C. diff* to others?

If you are infected, you can spread the disease to others. However, only people who are hospitalized or on antibiotics are likely to become ill. For safety precautions, you should do the following to reduce the chance of spreading *C. diff* to others:
- Wash your hands with soap and water, especially after using the restroom and before eating.

(continued)

Figure 4-16. *Clostridium difficile* Fact Sheet, *continued*

- Clean surfaces in bathrooms, kitchens, and other areas on a regular basis with household detergent/disinfectants.

What should I do if I think I have *C. diff* disease?
See your healthcare provider.

This fact sheet can be used as a tool to help educate patients who are at risk for C. diff.

Source: Centers for Disease Prevention and Control. Available at http://www.cdc.gov/ncidod/dhqp/id_CdiffFAQ_general.html (accessed Dec. 2, 2009).

- If you are overweight, talk to your doctor about a diet plan to help you lose excess weight before surgery.
- If you are diabetic, closely monitor your blood-glucose levels prior to surgery, and give your surgeon a written report of your results.
- Do not shave the surgical site. Shaving can leave nicks in the skin for bacteria to enter. Some organizations also recommend that women do not shave their legs or underarms for one week prior to the surgery due to an increased risk for infection at other sites.
- The night before and the morning of surgery, bathe with chlorhexidine.
- Choose a surgeon with a low infection rate for your type of procedure. Ask the surgeon about his or her infection rates.
- Ask your doctor about keeping you warm during surgery.
- On the day of your surgery, remind your doctor or nurse that you may need an antibiotic one hour before the first incision.

After Surgery

Patients should be taught to take the following steps after surgery to help prevent SSIs[33–35]:
- Wash hands thoroughly after using the bathroom.
- Remind doctors and nurses to clean their hands before treating you.
- Ask family and other visitors to wash their hands well.
- Do not touch or attempt to adjust surgical dressings until instructed to do so.

Figure 4-17. *Clostridium Difficile* Brochure

Questions?

_____
_____
_____
_____
_____
_____
_____
_____
_____
_____
_____
_____
_____
_____
_____
_____
_____
_____

Please ask your nurse
Or doctor if you have any
Questions.

Bethesda Health Group
Form # 8870-427-GR-B-D-PA 5/08

**Clostridium
Difficile
(C. difficile)**

The Bethesda Staff
hopes that you find the
following information
helpful during your
stay. Please ask your
nurse or doctor if you
have any questions,
Thank You.

This brochure can help staff members educate patients and families about preventing the spread of C. difficile.

(continued)

**For a downloadable version of this figure, please go to
http://www.jcrinc.com/NRIC09/Extras/.**

- Keep the skin around intravenous (IV) catheters and surgical dressings clean and dry; notify the nurse if a dressing becomes loose, wet, or soiled.
- Ask friends and family members not to visit if they feel ill.
- Notify your doctor (or other designated health care worker) if you note any of the following[36]:
  - Pain or tenderness
  - Increase in pus or other drainage from the wound
  - Foul odor from the wound
  - Swelling at the surgical site
  - Redness or darker skin around the wound

Figure 4-17. *Clostridium Difficile* Brochure, *continued*

What is C. Difficile?

Clostridium Difficile (C.Difficile) is a bacteria tha produces a toxin (a type of poison) that can cause an inflammation of the large intestine also known as colitis.

What are the symptoms of C.Difficile?

Common symptoms include diarrhea, fever and abdominal pain. In some cases diarrhea may not occur. C. Difficile may or may not be present in stools.

Who gets C. difficile?

C. difficile can be part of the normal bacteria that live in the large intestine. It also can be acquired in the large intestine after a hospitalization. Taking antibiotics can change the normal balance of bacteria in your large intestine, making it easier for C. difficile to grow and cause the toxin to be produced. C. difficile has been found on the hands of persons and in the environment surrounding infected patients.

Is C. difficile treatable?

Mild diarrhea often resolves as soon as the antibiotics that caused the symptoms in the first place are no longer taken. More serious diarrhea can last longer without therapy.

- If C. difficile colitis is suspected, you may be asked to give a stool sample that will be tested for the toxin.

- C. difficile colitis is treatable with certain oral antibiotics like metronadazole (Flagyl) or Vancomycin.

- You and your visitors should pay particular attention to good hand washing.

Why are precautions needed?

Precautions are needed because surfaces like toilets and common areas that hands touch can become contaminated with the bacteria. The bacteria can live on surfaces for a long time if they are not properly cleaned. In order to prevent the spread to other residents it will be necessary for everyone to follow these precautions:

- You will need to take special care with hand washing. Ask you nurse for guidance in how to wash your hands properly. Hands must be washed after using the toilet or bed pan, before eating and leaving your room.

- It is also very important for all staff and visitors to wash their hands when they come in and leave your room. Do not be afraid to remind everyone to wash their hands. Washing hands with soap and water is more effective than use of alcohol based hand sanitizers.

- Staff will wear gowns and gloves if they expect to come in contact with stool (for example, with some toileting type procedures). Sometimes equipment, such as commodes, may be left in your room specifically for your use and will be cleaned & maintained by nursing staff.

- If you are ill with symptoms, you may be asked to remain in your room until symptoms subside.

Can I give C.difficile to my family or friends?

- Healthy people who are not taking antibiotics are at very low risk of developing colitis. Their best protection against even a small risk is to wash their hands after visiting you and follow the precautions. Other residents are at greater risk of getting C. difficile colitis.

- It is okay to hold, hug or kiss visitors or family members—even children and babies. Remember, good hand washing is the most important factor for preventing the spread of any germs.

Is there anything I need to report to the doctor or nurse?

You should tell your doctor or nurse if your symptoms return, for example diarrhea or fever

Bethesda Health Group
Form ## 8870-427-GR-B-D-PA 5/08

Source: Bethesda Health. Used with permission.

- Fever, chills, weakness
- Confusion
- Fast heartbeat
- Ask how they will follow up to monitor if a complication/infection develops later

Catheter-Associated Urinary Tract Infections

It is now well established that a major predisposing factor for health care–associated urinary tract infection is the presence of an indwelling urinary catheter.[37] Catheter-associated urinary tract infections (CAUTIs) are relatively common, because bacteria can easily enter the urethra from the drainage bag or the catheter entry site.[38]

Patients can do a number of things to help prevent CAUTIs if properly educated. Patients should be taught to do the following[38]:
- Wash hands before and after handling the catheter or drainage bag.
- Manipulate the catheter and catheter bag as little as possible; anchor the catheter to reduce movement or friction, which increases the risk of infection.
- Clean the insertion site daily with soap and water; dry thoroughly.
- Keep the drainage bag or catheter valve connected to the catheter at all times.
- Keep the drainage bag at a lower level than the body.
- Do not let the drainage bag touch the floor.
- Empty the drainage bag when it is full, if it is causing discomfort, or if it is pulling on the catheter.
- When inserting an intermittent catheter, use the lubricant provided by the health care provider.
- Wash reusable intermittent catheters after use according to the manufacturer's instructions.
- Contact your health care provider if you have symptoms of infection or if the catheter does not appear to be draining.

Central Line–Associated Bloodstream Infections

In today's medical practice, intravascular catheters are indispensable in many settings, including the home. Although intravascular catheters are necessary to provide vascular access, their use puts patients at risk for local and systemic infectious complications, including central line–associated bloodstream infections (CLABSIs).[39] The incidence of CLABSIs varies considerably by type of catheter, frequency of catheter manipulation, and patient-related factors (for example, underlying disease and acuity of illness).[39]

The most frequently used devices for vascular access are peripheral venous catheters.[39] Although the incidence of local or bloodstream infections associated with peripheral venous catheters is usually low, serious infectious complications produce considerable annual morbidity because of the frequency with which such catheters are used.[39]

Because central venous catheters are placed in major veins, serious infections can occur very quickly.[38] According to the Institute for Healthcare Improvement (IHI), nurses should teach their patients and their patients' families to do the following to help prevent CLABSIs[40]:
- Watch the hospital staff to make sure they wash their hands before and after working with you.

- Ask the doctors and nurses lots of questions before you agree to a line. Questions can include: Which vein will you use to put in the line? How will you clean the skin when the line goes in? What steps are you taking to lower the risk of infection? How long will I need the catheter?
- Make sure the doctors and nurses check the line every day for signs of infection. They should only replace the line when needed and not on a schedule. The catheter should be removed as soon as is feasible.

In today's health care environment, patients are frequently released from the hospital with central lines in place. The National Center for Clinical Excellence (NICE) suggests that nurses should teach their patients and their patients' families the following strategies to help prevent CLABSIs while at home[38]:

- Follow the instructions given by your health care worker at all times.
- Perform appropriate hand hygiene before touching the central venous catheter.
- Wear sterile gloves for touching the insertion site or changing the dressing.
- Change the dressing every seven days (sooner if it becomes wet, dirty, or loose).
- Clean the catheter and its entry points before and after use.
- Do not put any cream, ointment, or solution on the insertion site unless instructed by your health care provider.
- Contact your health care worker if signs of infection develop (fever, swelling, feeling unwell).

Nurses should provide patients and their families with an emergency number and instructions about when to call it, as well as a number to call during office hours if any problems should arise.[38]

Tools to Educate Patients and Families About CLABSIs

The following tools can help nurses educate patients and families about the prevention of CLABSIs:

- **Prevent Central Line–Associated Bloodstream Infections Fact Sheets.** Available in English and Spanish (*see* Figures 4-18, page 136, and 4-19, page 138).

Ventilator-Associated Pneumonia

Ventilator-associated pneumonia (VAP) is defined as pneumonia occurring in a person who is being assisted by mechanical ventilation.[41] Risk factors include the following[41]:

- Longer duration of mechanical ventilation

Figure 4-18. Prevent Central Line Infections: A Fact Sheet for Patients and Their Families (English Version)

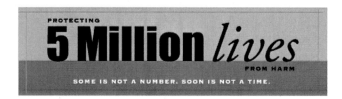

What You Need to Know about Central Line Infections (CLI):
A Fact Sheet for Patients and their Family Members

Patients who need frequent intravenous (IV) medications, blood, fluid replacement and/or nutrition may have a central venous catheter (or "line") placed into one of their veins. This line can stay in place for days and even weeks.

Catheter-related bloodstream infections (CR-BSI):

Lines are often very helpful. But sometimes they cause infections when bacteria grow in the line and spreads to the patient's bloodstream. This is called a "catheter-related bloodstream infection" (CR-BSI). It is very serious and 20 percent (or 1 out of 5) of patients who get CR-BSI die from it.

A bundle of 5 care steps to prevent CR-BSI:

Doctors and nurses can help prevent CR-BSI by using a bundle of 5 "care steps." Hospitals find that when all 5 of these steps are done that there are almost no cases of CR-BSI. The bundle of care steps are:
- Using proper hand hygiene. Everyone who touches the central line must wash their hands with soap and water or an alcohol cleanser.
- Wearing maximal barrier precautions. The person who inserts the line should be in sterile clothing – wearing a mask, gloves, and hair covering. The patient should be fully covered with a sterile drape, except for a very small hole where the line goes in.
- Cleaning the patient's skin with "chlorhexidine" (a type of soap) when the line is put in.
- Finding the best vein to insert the line. Often, this is the subclavian vein (in the chest) which is not as likely to get an infection as veins in the arm or leg.
- Checking the line for infection each day. The line should be taken out only when no longer needed and not on a schedule.

(continued)

This handout may help patients and family members assist in the prevention of CLABSIs.

Figure 4-18. Prevent Central Line Infections: A Fact Sheet for Patients and Their Families (English Version), *continued*

How patients and family members can help:

- Watch the hospital staff to make sure they wash their hands before <u>and</u> after working with the patient. Do not be afraid to remind them to wash their hands!
- Ask the doctors and nurses lots of questions before you agree to a line. Questions can include: Which vein will you use to put in the line? How will you clean the skin when the line goes in? What steps are you taking to lower the risk of infection?
- Make sure the doctors and nurses check the line every day for signs of infection. They should only replace the line when needed and not on a schedule.

Learn more about central line infections as they relate to the 5 Million Lives Campaign at www.ihi.org.

> **The 5 Million Lives Campaign** is an initiative to protect patients from five million incidents of medical harm over the next two years (December 2006 – December 2008).
>
> http://www.ihi.org/IHI/Programs/Campaign/Campaign.htm

Information provided in this Fact Sheet is intended to help patients and their families in obtaining effective treatment and assisting medical professionals in the delivery of care. The IHI does not provide medical advice or medical services of any kind, however, and does not practice medicine or assist in the diagnosis, treatment, care, or prognosis of any patient. Because of rapid changes in medicine and information, the information in this Fact Sheet is not necessarily comprehensive or definitive, and all persons intending to rely on the information contained in this Fact Sheet are urged to discuss such information with their health care provider. Use of this information is at the reader's own risk.

This document is in the public domain and may be used and reprinted without permission provided appropriate reference is made to the Institute for Healthcare Improvement.

Source: Institute for Healthcare Improvement. http://www.ihi.org/NR/ rdonlyres/6EC98A37-8B5E-4821-B0FE-DA1AB651D834/0/CentralLineInfectionsPtsandFam.pdf. Used with permission.

Figure 4-19. Prevent Central Line Infections: A Fact Sheet for Patients and Their Families (Spanish Version)

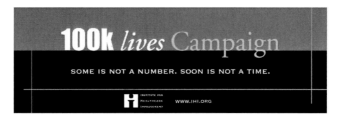

Lo Que Usted Debe Saber sobre Infecciones de las Vías Centrales: *Página de Informe para Pacientes y Sus Familiares*:

Para aquellos pacientes que necesitan frecuentes infusiones de medicamentos, sangre, o reemplazos líquidos o nutricionales por vía intravenosa, se les puede poner un catéter (o vía central) en una de las venas. Las vías intravenosas pueden permanecer en uso durante varios días o varias semanas.

Infecciones del torrente sanguíneo asociadas al catéter.

Las vías centrales por lo general son muy útiles. Pero a veces causan infección cuando la bacteria crece dentro de la vía y se riega por el torrente sanguíneo del paciente. A esto se le llama una infección del torrente sanguíneo asociadas al catéter. Es una condición muy seria y el 20 por ciento (1 de cada 5) de los pacientes con este tipo de infección muere a causa de la infección.

Un conjunto de 5 pasos a tomar para prevenir las infecciones del torrente sanguíneo por vía del catéter:

Los doctores y las enfermeras pueden ayudar a prevenir las infecciones del torrente sanguíneo asociadas al catéter siguiendo este conjunto de 5 pasos. Varios hospitales han comprobado que cuando llevan a cabo <u>todos</u> los 5 pasos, desaparecen casi por completo los casos de infecciones al torrente sanguíneo asociadas al catéter. El conjunto de pasos es el siguiente:

- Practicar la higiene de mano apropiada. Todo aquel que toca la vía central debe lavarse las manos con agua y jabón o con alcohol de mano.
- Usar las barreras de máxima precaución. La persona que pone la vía central debe usar ropa estéril – usar mascarilla, guantes, y un gorro para cubrir el cabello. El paciente debe estar cubierto por completo por el campo estéril, salvo por donde entra la línea.
- Limpiar la piel del paciente con "clorhexidina" (un tipo de jabón) cuando se pone la vía central.

Este documento es parte del dominio público y se puede usar y reproducir sin permiso con tal de que se mencione apropiadamente al Instituto para el Mejoramiento de la Salud (Institute for Healthcare Improvement).

(continued)

This handout may help patients and family members assist in the prevention of CLABSIs.

Figure 4-19. Prevent Central Line Infections: A Fact Sheet for Patients and Their Families (Spanish Version), *continued*

- Encontrar la mejor vena para la vía central. A menudo, eta es la vena subclavia (en el pecho) que es menos propensa a las infecciones, cuando se compara a las venas del brazo o la pierna.
- Examinar la vía central a diario para detectar cualquier infección. La vía debe sacarse solo cuando sea necesario y no a base de un horario.

Cómo los pacientes y sus familiares pueden ayudar:

- Observe al personal del hospital y asegure que se laven las manos antes y después de tocar al paciente. ¡No tema a recordarles que se laven las manos!
- Haga muchas preguntas a sus doctores y enfermeras antes de acordar a recibir una vía central. Puede preguntar: ¿Qué vena va a usar para la vía central? ¿Cómo va a limpiar la piel cuando ponga la vía? ¿Qué medidas está tomando para reducir el riesgo de una infección?
- Asegure que los doctores y enfermeras examinen la vía central todos los días para detectar cualquier señal de infección. La vía debe sacarse solo cuando sea necesario y no a base de un horario.

Puede aprender más acerca de infecciones de las vías centrales con relación a la Campaña para Salvar 100.000 Vidas en el siguiente sitio web www.ihi.org.

La Campaña para Salvar 100.000 Vidas es un esfuerzo nacional del Instituto para el Mejoramiento de la Salud (Institute for Healthcare Improvement) creado para involucrar y comprometer a más de 2.600 hospitales americanos a implementar cambios en el cuidado médico que han resultado exitosos en la prevención de las muertes evitables. La meta de la Campaña es de salvar 100.000 vidas para junio del 2006.

http://www.ihi.org/IHI/Programs/Campaign/Campaign.htm

La información que aparece en esta hoja se provee con la intención de ayudar a pacientes y a sus familiares a recibir buen cuidado médico y para asistir a los profesionales médicos a prestar cuidado médico. El Instituto para el Mejoramiento de la Salud no da consejos médicos ni presta servicios médicos de ninguna clase, y no práctica medicina ni asiste en el diagnóstico, tratamiento, cuidado, o prognosis de ningún paciente. A causa de los rápidos cambios en la medicina y la información, la información en esta hoja no pretende estar completa ni tampoco es definitiva. Toda persona con la intención de usar la información contenida en esta hoja, debe consultar con su proveedor médico. El uso de esta información es a su propio riesgo.

Este documento es parte del dominio público y se puede usar y reproducir sin permiso con tal de que se mencione apropiadamente al Instituto para el Mejoramiento de la Salud (Institute for Healthcare Improvement).

Source: Institute for Healthcare Improvement. http://www.ihi.org/NR/rdonlyres/ 6EC98A37-8B5E-4821-B0FE-DA1AB651D834/0/CentralLineInfectionsPtsandFam_Spanish_.pdf. Used with permission.

- Advanced age
- Depressed level of consciousness
- Preexisting lung disease
- Immune suppression from disease or medication
- Malnutrition
- Frequency of oral care when the patient is being ventilated or is on the ventilator

When someone is gravely ill, the patient and/or family may have to decide whether to have the patient placed on a ventilator. This decision can be very difficult.[42] However, in some cases, the use of a ventilator is a quality-of-life decision. For some people, staying alive via mechanical ventilation is not acceptable.[42]

Some patients make their wishes known in advance through advanced directives. But even with the best advanced planning, patients and family members often must make decisions in crisis situations.[42] Because each illness is different, being well informed about the patient's illness and the risks associated with mechanical ventilation can help with the decision-making process.[42] Nurses can help by providing this education. When patients and families know what the choices and consequences are, they can better make decisions that are consistent with the patient's wishes and values.[42]

If the decision is made to place the patient on a ventilator, nurses should encourage patients and family members to ask the following questions to help prevent VAP[43]:
- Are you going to raise the head of the bed when [patient] is on the ventilator? Raising the head of the bed helps prevent aspiration, a common cause of VAP.
- How are you going to prevent stomach ulcers? People on ventilators are prone to stress ulcers, so peptic ulcer disease prophylaxis is recommended.
- What will you do to prevent blood clots? People who are immobile for long periods of time are at risk for deep vein thrombosis (DVT), so DVT prophylaxis is recommended.
- When can [patient] try breathing on his or her own? Patients who receive mechanical ventilation for long periods of time are at increased risk of VAP.

Tools for Educating Family Members About Ventilator-Associated Pneumonia
The following tools can help nurses educate family members about VAP:
- **JAMA Patient Page: Ventilator-Associated Pneumonia.** Available at http://jama.ama-assn.org/cgi/content/full/300/7/864?etoc.

- **Prevent Ventilator-Associated Pneumonia Fact Sheets.** Available in English and Spanish (*see* Figures 4-20, page 142, and 4-21, page 144).

Food Safety

Each year, millions of illnesses in the United States are caused by foodborne bacteria.[44] According to the U.S. Food and Drug Administration (FDA), approximately 2% to 3% of all foodborne illnesses lead to secondary long-term illnesses. For example, certain strains of *Escherichia coli* can cause kidney failure in young children and infants.[44]

Common symptoms of foodborne illness include diarrhea, abdominal cramps, fever, headache, and vomiting.[45] These symptoms can develop as early as 30 minutes after eating contaminated food or as late as two weeks after consumption.[45]

Nurses should be knowledgeable about food safety and should educate patients about each step in the food-handling process—from shopping to storing leftovers and eating out.[45] The following information can help nurses educate patients about food safety.

Hand Hygiene

Germs can be transmitted from unclean hands to food, usually by an infected food preparer who did not wash his or her hands after using the toilet, touched contaminated surfaces before handling food, or otherwise handled food improperly.[46] The germs are then passed to those who eat the food. Germs can also be transmitted from raw, uncooked foods, such as chicken, to hands; the germs are then transferred to other foods, such as salad. Cooking the raw food kills the initial germs, but the salad remains contaminated.[46]

Cross-Contamination

Cross-contamination occurs when harmful bacteria are transferred to food from other foods, cutting boards, utensils, and so forth if they are not handled properly. This is especially true when handling raw meat, poultry, and seafood. The U.S. Department of Agriculture's (USDA) International Food Safety Council developed the following steps to help consumers prevent cross-contamination and reduce the risk of foodborne illness[47]:

- When shopping, separate raw meat, poultry, and seafood from other foods in your shopping cart. Place these foods in plastic bags to prevent their juices from dripping onto other foods.

Figure 4-20. Prevent Ventilator-Associated Pneumonia: A Fact Sheet for Patients and Their Families (English Version)

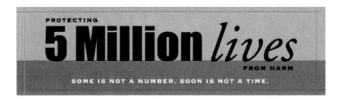

What You Need to Know about Ventilator-Associated Pneumonia (VAP): *A Fact Sheet for Patients and their Family Members*

Ventilator-Associated Pneumonia (VAP) is a lung infection that can happen to patients who are on ventilators (machines to help them breathe). This infection is very serious. About 15 percent (1 or 2 out of 10) of patients on ventilators get VAP. About half (50 out of 100) the patients with VAP die from it.

Some hospital patients need help breathing, either because they have just had a major operation or because they are very ill. These patients are often placed on a ventilator, a machine that supplies regular breaths through a tube inserted in the patient's mouth, nose, or through a hole in the front of the neck. Most of these patients recover, and the ventilator can be removed. However, there are proven ways to help prevent VAP – and patients and families can help to make sure these things are done.

A bundle of 4 care steps to prevent VAP:

Doctors and nurses can help prevent VAP by using a bundle of 4 "care steps." Hospitals find that when all 4 of these steps are done that there are almost no cases of VAP. The bundle of care steps are:
- Raising the head of the patient's bed between 30 and 40 degrees.
- Giving the patient medication to prevent stomach ulcers.
- Preventing blood clots when patients are lying very still.
- Seeing if patients can breathe on their own when waking up after surgery.

This document is in the public domain and may be used and reprinted without permission provided appropriate reference is made to the Institute for Healthcare Improvement.

(continued)

This handout may help family members feel empowered to ask questions that may help prevent VAP or complications of VAP.

Figure 4-20. Prevent Ventilator-Associated Pneumonia: A Fact Sheet for Patients and Their Families (English Version), *continued*

How family members can help:

Ask the nurses and doctors these questions:
- Are you going to raise the head of the bed when [patient] is on the ventilator?
- How are you going to prevent stomach ulcers?
- What will you do to prevent blood clots?
- When can [patient] try breathing on his or her own?

Learn more about ventilator-associated pneumonia as it relates to the 5 Million Lives Campaign on www.ihi.org.

The 5 Million Lives Campaign is an initiative to protect patients from five million incidents of medical harm over the next two years (December 2006 – December 2008).

http://www.ihi.org/IHI/Programs/Campaign/Campaign.htm

Information provided in this Fact Sheet is intended to help patients and their families in obtaining effective treatment and assisting medical professionals in the delivery of care. The IHI does not provide medical advice or medical services of any kind, however, and does not practice medicine or assist in the diagnosis, treatment, care, or prognosis of any patient. Because of rapid changes in medicine and information, the information in this Fact Sheet is not necessarily comprehensive or definitive, and all persons intending to rely on the information contained in this Fact Sheet are urged to discuss such information with their health care provider. Use of this information is at the reader's own risk.

This document is in the public domain and may be used and reprinted without permission provided appropriate reference is made to the Institute for Healthcare Improvement.

Source: Institute for Healthcare Improvement. http://www.ihi.org/NR/rdonlyres/ 818C1992-F318-4DBD-AE54-B45BCD3AD7DB/0/VentilatorAssociatedPneumonia PatandFamSheet.pdf. Used with permission.

Figure 4-21. Prevent Ventilator-Associated Pneumonia: A Fact Sheet for Patients and Their Families (Spanish Version)

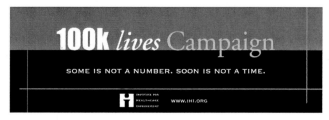

Lo Que Usted Debe Saber sobre la Neumonía Asociada a la Ventilación Mecánica (NAV):
Página de Informe para Pacientes y Sus Familiares:

La Neumonía Asociada a la Ventilación Mecánica (NAV) es una infección del pulmón que puede ocurrir cuando un paciente está conectado a un ventilador (una máquina que ayuda al paciente a respirar). Esta infección es muy seria. La NAV afecta a Aproximadamente el 15 por ciento (1 o 2 de cada 10) de los pacientes conectados a un respirador. La mitad (50 de 100) de esos pacientes con la NAV muere a causa de la infección.

Algunos pacientes necesitan ayuda para respirar, ya sea porque acaban de salir de una gran operación o porque están muy enfermos. A estos pacientes se les conecta a un respirador, una máquina que lleva oxígeno regularmente, por vía de sondas/tubos dentro de la boca, la nariz, o por un agujero al frente del cuello. La mayor parte de estos pacientes se recuperan y el respirador deja de ser necesario. Sin embargo, hay maneras efectivas para prevenir la NAV y los pacientes y familiares pueden ayudar a asegura que se tomen estas medidas.

Un conjunto de 4 pasos a seguir para prevenir la NAV:

Los doctores y las enfermeras pueden ayudar a prevenir la NAV siguiendo este conjunto de 4 pasos. Varios hospitales han comprobado que cuando llevan a cabo todos los 4 pasos, desaparecen casi por completo los casos de NAV. El conjunto de pasos es el siguiente:
- Elevar la cabeza del paciente ente 30-40 grados.
- Dar al paciente medicamento para prevenir las úlceras del estómago
- Prevenir coágulos cuando el paciente esta acostado y no tiene mucho movimiento
- Ver si el paciente puede respirar por si solo/sola cuando se despierta después de la cirugía

Este documento es parte del dominio público y se puede usar y reproducir sin permiso con tal de que se mencione apropiadamente al Instituto para el Mejoramiento de la Salud (Institute for Healthcare Improvement).

(continued)

This handout may help family members feel empowered to ask questions that may help prevent VAP or complications of VAP.

Figure 4-21. Prevent Ventilator-Associated Pneumonia: A Fact Sheet for Patients and Their Families (Spanish Version), *continued*

Cómo sus familiares pueden ayudar:

Haga estas preguntas a los médicos y enfermeras:
- ¿Va a elevar la cabeza del paciente cuando este conectado al respirador?
- ¿Cómo va a prevenir las úlceras del estómago?
- ¿Qué medidas va a tomar para prevenir coágulos de sangre?
- ¿Cuándo va a permitir al paciente a tratar de respirar por si solo/sola?

Puede aprender más acerca de la Neumonía Asociada a la Ventilación Mecánica (NAV) con relación a la Campaña para Salvar 100.000 Vidas en el siguiente sitio web www.ihi.org.

La Campaña para Salvar 100.000 Vidas es un esfuerzo nacional del Instituto para el Mejoramiento de la Salud (Institute for Healthcare Improvement) creado para involucrar y comprometer a más de 2.600 hospitales americanos a implementar cambios en el cuidado médico que han resultado exitosos en la prevención de las muertes evitables. La meta de la Campaña es de salvar 100.000 vidas para junio del 2006.

http://www.ihi.org/IHI/Programs/Campaign/Campaign.htm

La información que aparece en esta hoja se provee con la intención de ayudar a pacientes y a sus familiares a recibir buen cuidado médico y para asistir a los profesionales médicos a prestar cuidado médico. El Instituto para el Mejoramiento de la Salud no da consejos médicos ni presta servicios médicos de ninguna clase, y no práctica medicina ni asiste en el diagnóstico, tratamiento, cuidado, o prognosis de ningún paciente. A causa de los rápidos cambios en la medicina y la información, la información en esta hoja no pretende estar completa ni tampoco es definitiva. Toda persona con la intención de usar la información contenida en esta hoja, debe consultar con su proveedor médico. El uso de esta información es a su propio riesgo.

Este documento es parte del dominio público y se puede usar y reproducir sin permiso con tal de que se mencione apropiadamente al Instituto para el Mejoramiento de la Salud (Institute for Healthcare Improvement).

Source: Institute for Healthcare Improvement. http://www.ihi.org/NR/rdonlyres/818C1992-F318-4DBD-AE54-B45BCD3AD7DB/0/VentilatorAssociatedPneumoniaPatandFam_Spanish_.pdf. Used with permission.

- When refrigerating food, place raw meat, poultry, and seafood in containers or sealed plastic bags to prevent their juices from dripping onto other foods. Store eggs in their original carton, and refrigerate as soon as possible.
- Wash hands with soap and hot water before and after handling food and after using the bathroom, changing diapers, or handling pets.
- Use hot, soapy water and paper towels or clean cloths to wipe up kitchen surfaces or spills. Wash cloths often in the hot cycle of your washing machine.
- Wash cutting boards, dishes, and countertops with hot, soapy water after preparing each food item and before you go on to the next item.
- Always use a clean cutting board. If possible, use one cutting board for fresh produce and a separate one for raw meat, poultry, and seafood.
- Always marinate food in the refrigerator, not on the counter. Sauce that is used to marinate raw meat, poultry, or seafood should not be used on cooked foods unless it is boiled just before using.
- When serving food, always use a clean plate. Never place cooked food back on the same plate or cutting board that previously held raw food.

Refrigeration

At room temperature, harmful bacteria in food can double in number every 30 to 40 minutes.[48] The more bacteria present, the greater the chance that a person can become sick.

The FDA recommends that consumers be taught the following rules for food refrigeration and thawing[48]:
- Refrigerate food quickly, because cold temperatures keep most harmful bacteria from multiplying. Hot food will not harm your refrigerator.
- Set your refrigerator no higher than 40°F (4°C) and your freezer at 0°F (–18° C). Check the temperature occasionally with an appliance thermometer.
- Refrigerate or freeze perishables, prepared food, and leftovers within two hours. Use refrigerated foods within four days. Most foods can be frozen indefinitely, but check for odor after defrosting.
- Divide large amounts of leftovers into shallow containers for quick cooling in the refrigerator.
- Do not pack the refrigerator too full. Cold air must circulate to keep food safe.
- At family outings or barbecues, use a cooler to keep perishable foods cold. Always use ice or cold packs, and fill your cooler to the top. A full cooler will maintain its cold temperatures longer than one that is partially filled.

- Never thaw foods at room temperature. Thaw food in the refrigerator or by immersing it in cold water. Change the water every half hour to keep the water cold.
- It is okay to thaw food in the microwave, but be sure to cook the food immediately after it is thawed.

Cooking

Food safety experts agree that foods are properly cooked when they are heated for a long enough time and at a high enough temperature to kill harmful bacteria that cause foodborne illness. This temperature can vary from one type of food to another. The FDA has developed the following tips to help consumers cook food safely[49]:

- Use a clean food thermometer to determine when food is done.
- Cook ground beef to at least 160°F (71°C).
- Cook roasts and steaks to an internal temperature of at least 145°F (63°C). Poultry should be cooked to a *minimum* internal temperature of 165°F (74°C).
- Cook fish until it is opaque and flakes easily with a fork.
- Cook eggs until the yolks and whites are firm. Do not use recipes that contain raw or partially cooked eggs unless you use pasteurized eggs.
- Leftovers should be reheated to 165°F (74°C). Bring sauces, soups, and gravies to a boil.

Food Safety When Eating Out

Many people eat out these days, so it is important that they be educated about food safety when eating in restaurants. The FDA has developed the following tips for consumers to follow when eating in restaurants[50]:

- If the restaurant does not look clean to you, eat somewhere else.
- Always order your food fully cooked, especially meat, poultry, fish, and eggs. When your hot meal arrives, make sure it is hot and thoroughly cooked before you eat it. If it is not, send it back.
- Do not eat eggs that are raw or not fully cooked. These can be hidden in salads, custards, and some sauces.
- Do not eat raw oysters.
- Be careful with leftovers. If you will not be home within two hours, leave the leftovers behind.
- Take your leftovers home right away, and put them in the refrigerator.

Medications

Patients can do a number of things to prevent infection when self-administering medications. Nurses should provide patients with the following safety tips[51,52]:

- Thoroughly wash hands before and after administering medications.
- If using a medication that requires a multiuse medication cup, wash the cup thoroughly between uses.
- Wash pill organizers frequently. A good rule of thumb is to wash before refilling.
- If using medication that requires a dropper, make sure the dropper tip is not chipped or cracked; do not touch the dropper tip to your eye, ear, nose, or anything else.
- When using eyedrops, immediately replace and tighten the cap after use. Do not wipe or rinse the dropper tip.
- When using ear or nose drops, clean the dropper tip with warm water after each use, then immediately replace and tighten the cap.
- When administering an injection, swab the injection site or IV port with alcohol. After removing the needle cap, do not touch the needle to any surface except what is necessary to draw the medication into the syringe and to give the injection (for example, rubber stopper of vial, inside of ampoule, injection site, or port). Discard used needles in a hazardous waste container for needles. Do not recap the needle.
- When using an inhaler, hold the inhaler one to two inches from the mouth, or use a spacer. If using a steroid inhaler, rinse mouth after each use. Soak the inhaler case and spacer in warm water and a mild clear detergent once a week. Rinse, then allow to air dry on a paper towel.

Pet Safety

Many studies have demonstrated the health benefits of owning a pet,[53] but pets can also cause infection, particularly in children, the elderly, and people who are immunocompromised.[54] Exotic pets, such as birds or reptiles, pose the greatest risk, but dogs and cats can also cause infectious diseases in humans.[54] Patients who own pets should be taught to take the following precautions to avoid infection[53,55,56]:

- If your pet has a wound that is not healing, have it checked by a veterinarian. This could be a sign of MRSA, which can be passed from animals to humans.
- Wash your hands after petting your animal.
- Make sure your pet's vaccinations are current.
- Do not feed pets raw meat.

- Have your pet's feces checked for worms at least annually.
- Keep cages and pens clean.
- Do not use pet waste as fertilizer.
- Do not change the litter box or bird cage if you are pregnant.
- Wear gloves when changing the litter box; change cat litter daily.
- Keep your pet's nails trimmed to avoid scratches.
- Keep your pet clean and well-groomed.
- Perform oral hygiene for cats and dogs.
- If you are immunocompromised, avoid cleaning tanks for amphibians and fish.

Discharge Planning

Discharge planning should begin well in advance of the patient's discharge, possibly even as early as admission. Discharge planning includes educating the patient and family about infection prevention and control as it relates to the patient's diagnosis and condition. It also includes conducting a lifestyle and home assessment. In addition, the patient should be assessed for his or her decision-making ability and ability to comprehend discharge instructions.[57]

When preparing a patient for discharge, the nurse, in collaboration with the case manager and social worker, should ascertain whether the patient has physical barriers to continuing care, such as lack of transportation to follow-up appointments or lack of appropriate equipment or supplies at home.[57] If the patient needs assistance with transportation or equipment needs, referrals should be made to community-based agencies that provide the necessary resources or services.[58] Home health care should also be arranged, if warranted.[58]

If a patient is being transferred to another facility, the nurse should contact the receiving facility and discuss the patient's plan of care and any follow-up measures that will be necessary to meet the patient's ongoing needs. A written discharge summary and current medication list should also be sent to the receiving facility.

Prior to discharge, the nurse and the patient should discuss the following[58]:
- The patient's current condition.
- Any potential symptoms, problems, or changes that may occur after release from care and what to do if these occur.
- Medications that the patient will be taking and any potential interactions or side effects. The patient should be given a written medication list with specific

instructions about how to take each medication and information about possible side effects. The nurse should then ask the patient to demonstrate how to take the medications.

- Signs and symptoms of infection.
- Who to call if questions or problems arise.

Early planning can help ensure a smooth transition from one level of care to the next. Careful planning and patient education can help prevent infection after discharge or control the spread of infection once the patient is no longer in a controlled environment.

References

1. Pugliese G.: Infection control is everybody's business—People and opinions. *Healthcare Purchasing News.* Sept. 2002. http://findarticles.com/p/articles/mi_m0BPC/is_/ai_91653597 (accessed Jan. 8, 2009).
2. Pittet D., Donaldson L.: Challenging the world: Patient safety and health care–associated infection. *Int J Qual Health Care* 18:4–8, Feb. 2006.
3. Centers for Disease Control and Prevention: *2007 Guideline for Isolation Precautions: Preventing Transmission of Infectious Agents in Healthcare Settings.* http://www.cdc.gov/ncidod/dhqp/pdf/guidelines/Isolation2007.pdf (accessed Jun. 25, 2009).
4. The Best Illness Prevention: Hand Washing. *Adv Nurse Pract.* 2004. http://nurse-practitioners.advanceweb.com/sharedresources/advancefornp/resources/downloadableresources/np030104_p76handout.pdf (accessed Jan. 8, 2009).
5. Joint Commission Resources: Educating patients about infection control: Complying with NPSG.13.01.01. *Joint Commission Perspectives on Patient Safety* 8:10–11, Sep. 2008.
6. McGuckin M., Waterman R., Shubin A.: Consumer attitudes about healthcare-acquired infections and hand hygiene. *Am J Med Qual* 21:342–346, Sep.–Oct. 2006.
7. Centers for Disease Control and Prevention: *An Ounce of Prevention Keeps the Germs Away: Seven Keys to a Safer Healthier Home.* http://www.cdc.gov/ounceofprevention/docs/oop_brochure_eng.pdf (accessed Jan. 8, 2009).
8. Joint Commission Resources: Risk management. Patient isolation: Putting patients at risk? *Joint Commission Perspectives on Patient Safety* 4:7–8, Jun. 2004.
9. Parker L.: Infection control: Maintaining the personal hygiene of patients and staff. *Br J Nurs* 13:474–478, Apr.–May 2004.
10. Murphy S.L., et al.: Bath transfers in older adult congregate housing residents: Assessing the person-environment interaction. *J Am Geriatr Soc* 54:1265–1270, Aug. 2006.
11. Gill T.M., Han L., Allore H.G.: Bath aids and the subsequent development of bathing disability in community-living older persons. *J Am Geriatr Soc* 55:1757–1763, Nov. 2007.
12. London F.: Teaching patients about wound care. *Home Healthc Nurse* 25:497–500, Sep. 2007.

13. Michigan Department of Community Health, Michigan Antibiotic Resistance Reduction Coalition: *MRSA: What You Should Know.* 2006. http://www.michigan.gov/documents/MRSA_brochure_FINAL_167898_7.pdf (accessed Apr. 8, 2009).

14. Missouri PRO: *Prepare for Your Surgery.* Jun. 2003. http://www.ihi.org/NR/rdonlyres/3673BFD6-2903-45C9-8052-D7E9B865660F/547/sip_ptbrochure_MOQIO_7SOW.pdf (accessed Apr. 8, 2009).

15. Centers for Disease Control and Prevention: *Influenza: The Disease.* http://www.cdc.gov/flu/about/disease/index.htm (accessed Sep. 8, 2009).

16. Centers for Disease Control and Prevention: *Key Facts About Seasonal Flu Vaccine.* http://www.cdc.gov/flu/protect/keyfacts.htm (accessed Sep. 8, 2009).

17. Patient Education Series: Influenza ("the flu"). *Nursing* 37:47, Oct. 2007.

18. Grota P.G.: Perioperative management of multidrug-resistant organisms in health care settings. *AORN* 86:361–368, quiz 369–372, Sep. 2007.

19. Archibald L.K., Banerjee S.N., Jarvis W.R.: Secular trends in hospital-acquired *Clostridium difficile* disease in the United States, 1987–2001. *J Infect Dis* 189(9):1585–1589, 2004.

20. McDonald L.C., Owings M., Jernigan D.B.: *Clostridium difficile* infection in patients discharged from U.S. short-stay hospitals, 1996–2003. *Emerg Infect Dis* 12(3):Internet serial, Oct. 2005. http://www.cdc.gov/ncidod/EID/vol12no03/pdfs/05-1064.pdf (accessed Jan. 15, 2009).

21. Joint Commission Resources: Case study: Preventing MRSA in the neonatal intensive care unit at Beth Israel Medical Center. *Joint Commission Perspectives on Patient Safety* 9:1–5, Jan. 2009.

22. Murillo J.L.: *Newborn MRSA Surveillance Questionnaire.* Newark, NJ: Newark Beth Israel Medical Center, 2008.

23. Institute for Healthcare Improvement: *Living with MRSA.* Mar. 2006. http://www.ihi.org/NR/rdonlyres/C70733CE-8C97-4BFE-880B-13322BD29B72/0/LivingwithMRSAHandbook.pdf (accessed Jan. 14, 2009).

24. Patient Education Series: How to keep family safe from your staph infection. *RN* 69:35, Feb. 2006.

25. Association for Professionals in Infection Control and Epidemiology: *MRSA.* http://www.preventinfection.org/AM/Template.cfm?Section=The_Superbug_MRSA&Template=/CM/HTMLDisplay.cfm&ContentID=10231 (accessed Jan. 14, 2009).

26. Centers for Disease Control and Prevention: *Information for the Public About VRE.* Apr. 2008. http://www.cdc.gov/ncidod/dhqp/ar_VRE_publicFAQ.html (accessed Feb. 5, 2009).

27. Vanderbilt Medical Center: *VRE.* http://www.mc.vanderbilt.edu/root/pdfs/infectioncontrol/VREOUTPT.DOC (accessed Feb. 5, 2009).

28. The Christ Hospital: *Patient Education for Vancomycin-Resistant Enterococcus (VRE).* Mar. 2008. http://www.thechristhospital.com/upload/docs/Departments/InfectionControl/Patient%20Education%20for%20VRE%20brochure%2028030.pdf (accessed Feb. 5, 2009).

29. Greenwich Hospital: *What Is VRE—Vancomycin Resistant Enterococci: Patient/Family Information Sheet.* http://www.greenhosp.org/pe_pdf/genmed_vre.pdf (accessed Feb. 5, 2009).

30. Joint Commission Resources: Minimizing the growing threat of *Clostridium difficile*. *Joint Commission Perspectives on Patient Safety* 6:5–6, Jun. 2006.

31. Lord C.: Preventing surgical-site infections after coronary artery bypass graft: A guide for the home health nurse. *Home Healthc Nurse* 24:28–35, quiz 36–37, Jan. 2006.

32. Runy L.A.: Infection control: They need to know. *Hosp Health Netw* 80:16, 18, Nov. 2006.

33. Preventing surgical site infections. *RN* 69:39, Aug. 2006.

34. Committee to Reduce Infection Deaths: *15 Steps You Can Take to Reduce Your Risk of a Hospital Infection.* http://www.hospitalinfection.org/protectyourself.shtml (accessed Jan. 9, 2009).

35. Joint Commission Resources: Preventing surgical site infections. *Joint Commission Perspectives on Patient Safety* 8:8–9, 11, Sep. 2008.

36. London F.: Teaching patients about wound care. *Home Healthc Nurse* 25:497–500, Sep. 2007.

37. Joint Commission Resources: Urinary catheter use at Spectrum Health hospitals. *The Source* 6:8, Jan. 2008.

38. National Institute for Clinical Excellence: *Prevention of Healthcare-Associated Infections in Primary and Community Care.* London, UK: National Institute for Clinical Excellence, 2003.

39. Centers for Disease Control and Prevention: *Overview of Intravascular Catheter-Related Bloodstream Infections.* Updated Sep. 27, 2005. http://www.cdc.gov/ncidod/dhqp/dpac_iv.html (accessed Jan. 17, 2009).

40. Institute for Healthcare Improvement: *What You Need to Know About Central Line Infections (CLI): A Fact Sheet for Patients and Their Family Members.* http://www.ihi.org/NR/rdonlyres/6EC98A37-8B5E-4821-B0FE-DA1AB651D834/0/CentralLineInfectionsPtsandFam.pdf (accessed Jan. 17, 2009).

41. Torpy J.M.: JAMA patient page: Ventilator-associated pneumonia. *JAMA* 300:864, Aug. 2008.

42. Family Caregiver Alliance: *End-of-Life Choices: Feeding Tubes and Ventilators.* http://www.caregiver.org/caregiver/jsp/content_node.jsp?nodeid=399 (accessed Jun. 25, 2009).

43. Institute for Healthcare Improvement: *Prevention of Ventilator-Associated Pneumonia.* http://www.ihi.org/NR/rdonlyres/35B687FE-D4D0-44E5-A671-E76D74BB8D9F/0/vap.pdf (accessed Jan. 15, 2009).

44. Partnership for Food Safety Education: *Foodborne Illness.* http://www.fightbac.org/content/view/7/8/ (accessed Jan. 29, 2009).

45. Partnership for Food Safety Education: *Foodborne Illness Info.* http://www.fightbac.org/content/view/27/52/ (accessed Jan. 29, 2009).

46. Centers for Disease Control and Prevention: *Why Is Handwashing Important?* http://www.cdc.gov/od/oc/media/pressrel/r2k0306c.htm (accessed Jan. 29, 2009).

47. U.S. Department of Agriculture Food Safety and Inspection Service/Food and Drug Administration Center for Food Safety and Applied Nutrition: *Be Smart. Keep Foods Apart. Don't Cross-Contaminate.* http://www.foodsafety.gov/~fsg/fs-apart.html (accessed Jan. 29, 2009).

48. U.S. Food and Drug Administration Center for Food Safety and Applied Nutrition National Science Teachers Association: *Food Safety for You! Chill.* http://www.cfsan.fda.gov/~dms/fttchill.html (accessed Jan. 29, 2009).

49. U.S. Food and Drug Administration Center for Food Safety and Applied Nutrition National Science Teachers Association: *Food Safety for You! Cook.* http://www.cfsan.fda.gov/~dms/fttcook.html (accessed Jan. 29, 2009).

50. U.S. Food and Drug Administration: *For Consumers: Restaurant and Take-Out Safety.* Updated May 1, 2009. http://www.fda.gov/ForConsumers/ByAudience/ForWomen/ucm118557.htm (accessed Jun. 25, 2009).

51. American Society of Health-System Pharmacists: *How to Administer.* http://www.safemedication.com/safemed/MedicationTipsTools/HowtoAdminister.aspx (accessed Jan. 29, 2009).

52. The Children's Medical Center: *Child Health Information: Metered-Dose Inhaler with/Without Spacer Device (MDI with Spacer).* http://www.childrensdayton.org/PDF_Files/childsafety/MDIWITHSPACER_1104.pdf (accessed Mar. 27, 2009).

53. Harvard University: Our pet causes. *Harvard Health Newsletter* pp. 6–7, Apr. 2008.

54. Harvard University: Infectious diseases: Living with germs. *Harvard Health Newsletter* p. 6, Feb. 2001.

55. Guay D.R.: Pet-assisted therapy in the nursing home setting: Potential for zoonosis. *Am J Infect Control* 29:178–186, Jun. 2001.

56. Kujubu D.A.: *Recommendations for Handling Pets in the ESRD Setting.* Updated Oct. 2007. http://www.ikidney.com/article.php?id=20071012011121 (accessed Feb. 11, 2009).

57. New York State Department of Health: *Discharge Planning.* Updated Sep. 2008. http://www.health.state.ny.us/professionals/patients/discharge_planning/index.htm (accessed Apr. 8, 2009).

58. National Alliance for Caregiving, United Hospital Fund of New York: *A Family Caregiver's Guide to Hospital Discharge Planning.* http://www.caregiving.org/pubs/brochures/familydischargeplanning.pdf (accessed Apr. 8, 2009).

Chapter 5

The Nurse's Role in Preventing and Controlling Infections in Special Settings and Populations

Infection prevention and control is problematic in most health care settings, and escalating rates of health care–associated infections (HAIs) are of concern for patients and health care professionals. Nurses in all settings should serve as good role models for patients and families and make sure they understand the basic principles of infection prevention and control. "As a consultant, I have observed a lot of people providing patient care," says Mary McGoldrick, M.S., R.N., C.R.N.I., home care and hospice consultant, Home Health Systems, Inc., a home health and hospice consulting firm in St. Simons Island, Georgia. "Normally, when they do something wrong, it's not intentional. Lack of knowledge and understanding contributes to breaches in infection control practices."

Different settings and different patient populations pose unique challenges to infection prevention and control. This chapter discusses those challenges and the nurse's role in preventing and controlling infections in the following settings and populations:
- Home care
- Ambulatory care
- Emergency department (ED)
- Maternity/neonatal units
- Pediatrics
- Oncology
- Long term care
- Behavioral health care

Home Care

With health care delivery shifting from acute care organizations to ambulatory, long term care, and community settings, it is more important than ever for home health nurses to be up-to-date on infection prevention and control practices.[1]

Although a wealth of knowledge about how to prevent and to control infections in the acute care setting is available, not as much information exists related to home care settings.[2] Infection prevention and control in the home care setting poses specific challenges for the home care nurse.[2]

According to McGoldrick, one of the difficulties with preventing and controlling infections in the home care setting is that the home care organization has no control over the home care environment. For example, the patient's home might be poorly sanitized, have inadequate plumbing, or have an insufficient climate control system.[2] "There is more environmental control in the hospital," says McGoldrick. "Sometimes in the home, there are rodents or other pests. There may also be a lack of refrigeration, electricity, or running water, although that's not as common. When you go to make that first site visit, you don't know what you'll be walking into."

Another major challenge for home health nurses is that the patient's home is far removed from other health care resources, so home care nursing is a largely autonomous practice, which leads to variations in practice.[3] Most home health nurses also do not have access to infection preventionists, and it is often difficult for them to get outside help if necessary.[3]

A lot of the focus on infection prevention and control in the home health setting should be on teaching the patient and family how to provide care, according to McGoldrick. "You're trying to teach people with different language skills and educational levels," she says. "They do the best they can to recall what they've been taught, but some types of care, such as infusion therapy, can be very complex. Show them what they can do to prevent infections. This could include hand-hygiene techniques, standard precautions, contact precautions, and/or how to perform dressing changes; it all depends on the patient's needs." As discussed in Chapter 4, teaching should include not only basic principles, such as hand hygiene, patient hygiene, and standard precautions, but also information about cleaning equipment and environmental surfaces and disposing of needles.

Cleaning Equipment and Environmental Surfaces

Some pathogens can survive for months on inanimate objects or environmental surfaces.[1] Therefore, patients need to be taught the importance of cleaning equipment and environmental surfaces, even if they do not appear soiled.[4,5] It is particularly important to keep surfaces clean in the kitchen and the bathroom.[4]

Cleaning and disinfecting surfaces and patient care equipment should be done on a regular basis, as defined by the home health agency.[5] Equipment used for patient care must be cleaned before it can be disinfected.[5] Cleaning can be done with soap and water. Disinfection should be done with an Environmental Protection Agency (EPA)—registered low—or intermediate-level disinfectant.[5]

In addition to instructing patients about the importance of cleaning and disinfecting equipment and environmental surfaces, it is equally important that home health staff be instructed to clean equipment between patients. This may include such items as stethoscopes, blood pressure cuffs, nursing bags, laptop computers, cell phones, and cameras.[1,5]

Disposing of Needles

Each year, nine million people will administer at least three billion injections in their own homes or in other public facilities.[6] Because improperly discarded needles can injure others or spread infection, it is important for home health nurses to instruct patients on proper methods for disposing of needles.[6] These may include the following[7]:

- Drop off or collection sites
- "Household hazardous waste" centers
- Residential "special waste" pickup services
- Syringe exchange programs
- Mail-back service
- Home needle destruction services

See Figure 5-1, page 158, for a patient education brochure detailing the above disposal methods.

Surveillance

Surveillance data available for infections that are acquired in the home are currently insufficient, so it is difficult to develop organism-specific prevention and

Figure 5-1. Protect Yourself, Protect Others: Safe Options for Home Needle Disposal

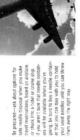

This brochure can help home health nurses educate their patients about safe needle disposal.

For a downloadable version of this figure, please go to http://www.jcrinc.com/NRIC09/Extras/.

(continued)

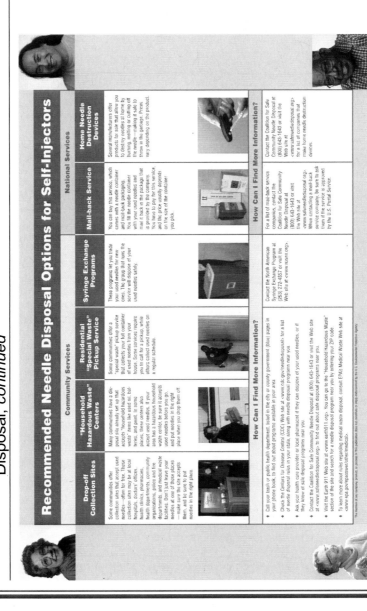

Figure 5-1. Protect Yourself, Protect Others: Safe Options for Home Needle Disposal, *continued*

Source: U.S. Environmental Protection Agency. Available at http://www.epa.gov/osw/nonhaz/industrial/medical/med-home.pdf (accessed Dec. 2, 2009).

intervention strategies.[3] It is therefore crucial for the home health nurse to assist in the data-collection process. "If the agency is collecting data on catheter-associated urinary tract infections, and you discover that your patient has a catheter-associated urinary tract infection, you should not only inform the physician in order to initiate treatment, but you should also report back to the home health agency," McGoldrick says. "If nurses are not properly reporting, the surveillance data won't be accurate."

Case Example:
Case Western University School of Nursing, Cleveland, Ohio

An infection control consultant at Case Western University School of Nursing in Cleveland, Ohio, conducted a study to determine whether nurses' bags might play roles in the spread of infection.[8] Four home health agencies were recruited to participate in the study. All nurses were asked to bring their bags to their next staff meetings but were not given an explanation as to why.[8] Although the nurses were given an opportunity to opt out of the study, most agreed to participate.[8]

Cultures were collected from the inside and the outside of the bags and from patient care equipment that was inside the bags.[8] A large percentage of the cultures collected from the bags themselves contained infectious agents. A smaller percentage of the equipment also tested positive for pathogens.[8] It was also determined that cloth bags contained more pathogens than leather bags.[8]

After the bags had been cleaned and then used for two weeks, the number of cultures that tested positive for pathogens in the first agency tested dropped by 31%.[8]

As a result of this study, the following recommendations were made to reduce the risk of spreading infection via the nurses' bags[8]:
• Standardize the type of bag that nurses are allowed to carry.
• Standardize cleaning protocols and cleaning solution.
• Clean nurse's bags weekly.
• Provide ongoing education to maintain awareness.

Ambulatory Care

Infections in the ambulatory setting can come from multiple sources. In addition to the risk of HAIs that are procedure- or treatment-related, reception and waiting areas in ambulatory facilities pose a risk for the spread of infectious diseases, such as measles, tuberculosis, and influenza.[9] "In ambulatory care, we're not only dealing with health care–associated infections and infections that are related to procedures," says Beverly Robins, field director, Division of Accreditation and Certification Operations, The Joint Commission, "but any communicable disease that is in the public realm."

According to Robins and Virginia McCollum, R.N., associate director, Standards Interpretation Group, The Joint Commission, early recognition and intervention are important parts of preventing and containing infections not only in the ambulatory setting but in any setting. In an ideal world, a patient with tuberculosis would not be allowed to enter an ambulatory facility, but that is not always the case.[9] Therefore, if someone is admitted to an ambulatory facility and is suspected to have tuberculosis, a mask should be immediately provided to that individual, and the patient should be referred to an appropriate treatment facility.[9] "If a patient comes in with tuberculosis, procedures, such as masking and isolating the patient and hand washing, need to be quickly implemented to prevent the infection from spreading," McCollum says.

Controlling Patient Flow and Patient Waiting Areas

Infection prevention and control in ambulatory care facilities should begin at the time the appointment is made.[9] For example, if a patient who is ill calls to make an appointment, the staff member who is scheduling the appointment should ask whether the patient has a rash or respiratory symptoms or whether he or she has had any recent exposure to a contagious illness.[9] Those who are suspected of having an infectious illness should be checked in immediately and moved to an exam room, thereby avoiding the waiting area.[9]

To limit the spread of infection in waiting areas, they should be designed as multiple small rooms instead of one large room, if possible.[9] This allows staff to separate patients with potentially contagious illnesses from those who are not ill (for example, patients with orthopedic injuries).[9]

Environmental Cleaning

All reusable equipment that comes in contact with the patient needs to be cleaned after each use.[9] "Surfaces need to be cleaned with appropriate disinfectants," Robins says. "Sometimes I observe staff wiping surfaces down, but they don't allow the

What Would You Do?

You are a nurse in an ambulatory clinic in an urban area where there has been a recent influenza outbreak. A man walks into the office and requests to see the doctor. The man looks very ill, is coughing into his hands, and has perspiration on his forehead. The waiting room is full of people who are waiting to see the doctor, and you fear the man may be contagious. What would you do?

In this scenario, it is likely that the patient has influenza, so it is important to get him away from the other patients before he gets close enough to spread infection or begins touching things in the waiting room. The nurse should give the patient a face mask, don a standard surgical mask to protect himself or herself from exposure to the patient's droplets, and escort the patient into an empty room. He or she should instruct the patient about respiratory etiquette and the importance of not touching anything while waiting for the physician. The nurse should then alert the doctor that the patient in that room is potentially infectious.

proper amount of time for the disinfecting solution to work. They need to make sure they are following the manufacturer's instructions." Although infections are not generally spread by exam-room furniture, the examination table should be covered with disposable paper or linen and changed between patients.[9]

"Staff need to use proper sterilization and storage techniques for surgical equipment," says McCollum. Packs that have been sterilized need to be appropriately identified before storing.[9] Autoclaves should be serviced on an annual basis, and the inner components should be taken out and cleaned regularly, then refilled with distilled water.[10]

Maintaining Asepsis

Maintaining asepsis during procedures is an important part of infection prevention and control in ambulatory facilities. If aseptic technique is followed at all times, the likelihood of bloodstream infections is decreased.[11] For example, the use of a full body drape when inserting a catheter creates maximum barrier sterility.[11] The risk for a patient developing a urinary tract infection (UTI) is also decreased if staff perform appropriate hand hygiene, don sterile gloves, and use sterile technique for urinary catheter insertion.[11]

Surveillance

"Nurses need to be current on issues related to communicable diseases within their communities and within their ambulatory care setting," McCollum says. "Ambulatory facilities need to have a designated person in charge of infection prevention and control. That person should be receiving alerts from public health officials about infectious diseases and be able to respond to the situation at hand. For example, before SARS [severe acute respiratory syndrome] hit the news, many ambulatory settings already had masks, gowns, and gloves ready and had educated their staff in advance."

Case Example:
Spivey Station Surgery Center, Jonesboro, Georgia

Spivey Station Surgery Center in Jonesboro, Georgia, has done a number of things to prevent and to control infection in its outpatient surgery center. One of its infection prevention initiatives was to standardize the use of only one chlorhexidine diacetate skin prep.[12] Prior to implementation, physicians were using approximately 50 different skin-prep products.[12]

Another method for preventing infection at Spivey Station was to clean the operating rooms daily.[12] This included removing all items from the room, wet vacuuming the walls, and cleaning all surfaces.[12]

A third method undertaken by Spivey Station for infection prevention was to organize the surgery center so that clean items come in on one side and dirty items go out on the other.[12]

Hand hygiene has also been an important part of Spivey Station's infection prevention program.[13] Staff members are required to tell patients when they are performing hand hygiene. Signs are also posted on all sinks that say, "Please make sure your care provider washes their hands today."[13]

Spivey Station follows patients up to 90 days to check for postoperative infections.[13] So far, the center has a zero infection rate.[13]

Emergency Department

One of the challenges that nurses face with regard to preventing and controlling infection in the ED is inadequate patient history of infection risks or previous exposure. Therefore, during triage, the nurse needs to ask patients about any rashes or skin lesions that are draining, or whether they have had fevers, diarrhea, recent exposures to someone with an infectious disease, recent hospital stays, or recent antibiotic therapies.[14] "When someone comes into the emergency department, you never know what risk they are for exposure or transmission," says Francine Westergaard, M.S.N., R.N., consultant for Joint Commission International and Joint Commission Resources. "It is important for nurses to question the patient or family about recent exposure to diseases, such as chicken pox, lice, pertussis, or tuberculosis. It is also important to determine if a patient has recently been on a trip out of the country, which may have resulted in an exposure to a communicable disease." If a patient answers, "yes" to any of the above questions, he or she should be put in isolation until further testing can be done.[14]

It is also important to triage patients who are arriving at the hospital via ambulance.[15] The nurse should ask the dispatcher if the patient has a respiratory illness with fever. If so, to prevent spreading germs throughout the ED, EMS workers should be instructed to leave the patient in the ambulance until hospital personnel gives them instructions about where to take the patient.[15] An N95 mask should be worn by all staff members who will be caring for the patient.[15]

Keeping Rooms and Equipment Clean

Another important aspect of infection prevention and control in the ED is ensuring that ED rooms and equipment are kept clean, even during high volume times. "Normally, when a patient is being transferred to a unit from the ED, housekeeping would be responsible for cleaning the ED room," Westergaard says. "In high volume situations, the nurse may be responsible, so it is important that nurses be educated about the appropriate methods for cleaning patient rooms, supplies, and equipment. Some viruses, such as RSV [respiratory syncytial virus], can live on a countertop for up to four hours. If a patient is transferred or discharged and the room is not cleaned appropriately and an immune-suppressed patient comes in, that patient is at high risk for exposure to the infection."

Equipment and surfaces in ED treatment rooms that should always be cleaned between patients include stretchers, mattresses, monitor cables, blood pressure cuffs, oxygen saturation probes, bedside tables, light switches, and door handles.[16]

Discharge Planning

Prior to discharge, in addition to teaching patients about hand hygiene, respiratory etiquette, wound care, and so forth (*see* Chapter 4), patients also need to be educated about when antibiotic therapy is appropriate and when it is not. "Many times, patients will come in with a virus, and the patient or parents will ask for antibiotics," says Westergaard. "It is the nurse's role to help patients and families understand why antibiotics won't help treat viral infections."

If an infectious patient is being discharged from the ED to another hospital unit or outpatient facility, it is also the nurse's responsibility to ensure that the receiving unit or facility is aware of the infection prior to discharge.[14] This is also important when sending a patient for inpatient services, such as radiology or laboratory services.[14]

Recognizing Infection Trends and Patterns

Nurses should be vigilant about looking for trends that may indicate a community outbreak. "If a nurse sees several patients from a community come in with common symptoms, he or she should question whether or not the hospital is experiencing an influx of patients that may be the beginning of an outbreak," Westergaard says. "The nurse should know when to contact the epidemiology department or to pull in other hospital support mechanisms."

Case Example:
Reducing Blood Culture Contamination Rates in the ED

An ED in a 963-bed community teaching hospital in northeastern Ohio conducted a study to compare blood culture–contamination rates in samples using a tincture of iodine skin prep to those using a newer skin prep product made of 2% chlorhexidine and 70% isopropanol.[17] For the first year of the study, all blood cultures were drawn in the ED using the tincture of iodine process. For the following year, all blood cultures were drawn using the following chlorhexidine/isopropanol process[17]:
1. Clean collection bottle top with an isopropyl alcohol pad.
2. Apply the chlorhexidine/isopropanol solution.

3. Use a back-and-forth motion to scrub the site vigorously for 30 seconds.
4. Allow 15 to 30 seconds for the skin to dry.
5. Perform venipuncture.

During year one of the study, 251 of 7,158 blood cultures (3.5%) were contaminated.[17] During year two, 169 of 7,606 (2.2%) were contaminated, a difference that was statistically significant.[17]

Maternity and Neonatal

Infection is a common cause of morbidity and mortality in neonatal intensive care units (NICUs).[18] Newborns, particularly preterm infants, are extremely vulnerable to infection. "One reason that infants are so vulnerable is that they haven't established their own immune systems yet," says Westergaard. Additionally, premature infants, particularly those with extremely low birth weights, often require ongoing intense medical therapies to sustain life.[18] "Premature infants frequently require medical technology to keep them alive," says Westergaard, "so we're sustaining life by connecting them to equipment that may introduce infections."

Infections can be introduced from mother to child during critical points in gestation or during vaginal delivery.[18,19] Recent literature has reported the occurrence of community-associated methicillin-resistant *Staphylococcus aureus* (MRSA) in postpartum women and neonates.[20] Outbreaks have also been reported in healthy, full-term newborns presenting with MRSA infection after discharge from normal newborn nurseries.[20] "In 1998, the first official report of MRSA in people with no known risk factors was released following the deaths of four children," says Jeremias Murillo, M.D., hospital epidemiologist, Newark Beth Israel Medical Center, Newark, New Jersey. "In the past, MRSA had always been associated with health care exposure. These were the first known cases of community-acquired MRSA. We now have more patients coming into the hospital already infected with MRSA. Some are chronic patients, but we're seeing an increasing number who have had no recent exposure to health care."

Bacterial infections are the most common cause of infant morbidity and mortality among low-birth-weight infants.[18] Early recognition and prompt initiation of antibiotic therapy can greatly improve outcomes.[18] "Nurses may be the first one contacted if the lab realizes there is a lab result that shows the baby has an infection," says Westergaard. "The nurse needs to disseminate this information to the other team members." NICU nurses should also have clear understandings of safety issues surrounding antibiotic use in neonatal populations, including indications for and contraindications for specific antibiotics prescribed on their units.

Health Care–Associated Infections in the NICU

Many sources of infection exist in the NICU environment. These include direct contact with infected caregivers; NICU overcrowding; contaminated respiratory equipment, incubators, or sinks; and contaminated blood products, parenteral nutrition solutions, and medication vials.[18] Nurses can help prevent and control infection by making sure equipment brought into patient-care areas is appropriately cleaned before and after each use and by using appropriate techniques for administering blood products, parenteral nutrition, and medications. Nurses should also help educate family members about infection prevention and control methods. "Nurses are the gate holders for infant safety," says Westergaard. "They are the ones responsible for teaching family members about infection prevention and control, including how and when to wash their hands and what precautions they need to take if the infant is in isolation. They also need to be taught what they should do to prevent the spread of infection if they become ill themselves."

Continuing Staff Education

Nurses and other caregivers have responsibilities to stay current with the latest evidence-based guidelines. "Advanced practice nurses and other nurse leaders should be disseminating this information to frontline staff and families," Westergaard says. "They are also the ones responsible for developing supporting policies and incorporating these practices into daily activities."

Case Example:
St. Luke's Children's Hospital, Boise, Idaho

In the spring of 2006, St. Luke's Children's Hospital in Boise, Idaho, saw an increase in the number of extremely low-birth-weight infants. As a result, it also saw an increase in the number of ventilator days and a rise in cases of ventilator-associated pneumonia (VAP).[21]

St. Luke's assembled a multidisciplinary team to tackle the problem. The team reviewed best practices and developed a performance improvement bundle.[21] The bundle consisted of best-practice standards related to hygiene (*see* Table 5-1, page 169), aspiration-prevention interventions (*see* Table 5-2, page 169), and preprinted orders (*see* Table 5-3, page 170).[21]

In the seven months following implementation of the performance-improvement bundle, St. Luke's had only one incidence of VAP.[21]

Pediatrics

Pediatric patients may pose some specific challenges when it comes to infection prevention and control. The variety of ages seen in pediatric health care settings requires that the nurse understand the age-based and developmental challenges for neonates, infants, toddlers, preschoolers, school-age, adolescent, and adult patients. According to Gail Potter-Bynoe, B.S., C.I.C., manager, Infection Prevention and Control, Children's Hospital Boston, viral infections are more common in the pediatric population and are also difficult to control. "Children have more infectious diseases and more that are contagious to others," says Potter-Bynoe. "Neonates and infants can be particularly vulnerable due to lack of immunization or incomplete immunization. With toddlers, there is a greater potential for exposure to and contamination of the environment due to lack of ability to control secretions and excretions. It is important that all health care workers are in tune to specific challenges based on the patient's age."

"In pediatrics, family-centered care presents unique challenges for infection prevention," Potter-Bynoe adds. "Parents and family members are actively involved in the care of their sick child, and potentially infected siblings are often with the family in the hospital."

In many hospitals, single-room isolation is used for children who are potentially infectious or highly susceptible to infection.[22] However, isolation nursing should only be used if it is necessary to protect patients, because in some cases, it may have serious psychological effects on the child and the family.[22]

Nurses can take the following steps to ensure that children on isolation and their family members do not feel alienated[22]:
• Educate patients and families about the need for isolation and how it works. This is why it is important for nurses to include families in education about infection prevention. "Families don't always understand the reasons for specific precautions

Table 5-1. Practice Standards for Reducing VAP: Hygiene

Increase emphasis on hand washing.

Use a new, sterile ET tube for each intubation attempt.

Wear gloves whenever handling the ventilator circuit.

Place a new orogastric tube for air evacuation every 7 days and with unplanned removals.

When repositioning patients, do not disconnect ventilator circuit from ET tube unless absolutely necessary.

Change ventilator circuit only when it is visibly soiled.

Change ventilator circuit after extubation and before reapplying circuit if extubation attempt does not succeed.

Source: Norris S.C., Barnes A.K., Roberts T.: When ventilator-associated pneumonias haunt your NICU—One unit's story. *Neonatal Netw* 28:59–66, Jan.–Feb. 2009. Used with permission.

Table 5-2. Practice Standards for Reducing VAP: Aspiration Prevention

Maintain the head of the bed at a 15- to 30-degree angle as tolerated. (We found that our open warmers could be raised to only 12 degrees.)

Use an oral sponge or sterile 2x2 gauze and sterile water to perform oral care every 4 hours as tolerated.

Suction oral cavity after oral care.

Use two different setups for oral and endotracheal suctioning; clearly label each one.

Do not use saline with suctioning except to clear suction catheter.

Drain water from ventilator circuit before turning patient.

Source: Norris S.C., Barnes A.K., Roberts T.: When ventilator-associated pneumonias haunt your NICU—One unit's story. *Neonatal Netw* 28:59–66, Jan.–Feb. 2009. Used with permission.

Table 5-3. Doctor's Orders and Progress Notes: NICU Ventilated Infant Protocol Orders

Increase emphasis on hand washing.

Use a new, sterile ET tube for each intubation attempt.

Wear gloves whenever handling the ventilator circuit.

Place a new orogastric tube for air evacuation every 7 days and with unplanned removals.

When repositioning patients, do not disconnect ventilator circuit from ET tube unless absolutely necessary.

Change ventilator circuit only when it is visibly soiled.

Change ventilator circuit after extubation and before reapplying circuit if extubation attempt does not succeed.

Source: Norris S.C., Barnes A.K., Roberts T.: When ventilator-associated pneumonias haunt your NICU—One unit's story. *Neonatal Netw* 28:59–66, Jan.–Feb. 2009. Used with permission.

or why there may be restrictions on the child's movements," Potter-Bynoe says. "With family-centered care, it's important to educate families on steps they can take to protect their child from health care–associated infections."

• Emphasize the value of visitors, but provide education. Many visitors may stay away if they do not understand isolation precaution techniques.

• Take time to talk to patients and families, and listen to any concerns.

• Suggest activities, such as television, radio, books, and newspapers.

• Give isolated patients and families rooms with windows when possible.

If it is not possible to isolate infectious patients, cohort nursing for children with the same infective organism is a potential alternative.[22]

Toys as a Potential Source of Infection

For hospitalized children, play can be a needed distraction that can help them cope and reduce pain and fear.[23] However, in one study conducted on a pediatric intensive care unit (PICU), 85% of the toys examined harbored viable bacteria.[23]

Nurses can do a number of things to ensure that toys are safe for use by children and to educate parents about infection prevention and control as it relates to the use of children's toys. These include the following[23]:

- If parents are bringing toys from home, encourage them to bring toys that can be easily disinfected.
- Discourage the practice of sharing toys between children.
- Clean visibly soiled toys as per organizational cleaning and disinfecting policy.
- Clean all toys periodically as per organizational cleaning and disinfecting policy.
- Encourage parents to take their child's toys home periodically or when visibly soiled for domestic washing.

Nurses as Infection Prevention Liaisons

Nurses can help prevent and control infections on pediatric units by acting as infection prevention liaisons. "At Children's Hospital Boston, we have unit-based liaisons who are trained in infection prevention and control and become the local experts for their floor," says Potter-Bynoe. "They field questions and identify issues that may need to be addressed. They may also act as flu ambassadors, giving out immunizations, or be involved in performance improvement projects, such as initiatives to reduce device-related infections."

Case Example: Hand-Washing Teaching Programs on Pediatric Intensive Care Units

A recent study was conducted on PICUs in Taiwan to determine whether a hand-washing video would improve the hand-washing skills of family members visiting patients in the PICU.[24] Study participants were split into two groups. One group viewed a hand-washing demonstration video that was specifically designed for this study and was then given an opportunity to ask questions. The other group did not view the video but was given the same information in the form of a poster presentation.[24]

Staff members recorded compliance with hand-washing policies as family members entered the unit. Accuracy of hand-washing technique was also recorded.[24] At the end of the study, compliance scores and scores for technique were significantly higher in the group that viewed the video than in the group that viewed the poster presentation.[24]

Oncology

Many oncology patients are at increased risk for infection; the risk of infection correlates with the degree of immunosuppression caused by the cancer and cancer-related treatment. Complications of infections are significant causes of morbidity and mortality in cancer patients.[25]

In addition to common pathogens, oncology patients may be at increased risk for opportunistic infection—that is, infection caused by pathogens that would normally not cause disease in people with healthy immune systems. "Patient-specific factors that increase the risk of infection include neutropenia, B- or T-cell deficiency, and/or disruption of skin or mucosal membranes as a result of surgery, chemotherapy, or radiation therapy," says Laura Zitella, R.N., M.S., N.P., A.O.C.N., nurse practitioner, Division of Oncology, Stanford University Cancer Center, Stanford, California. "Preventing infection in this high-risk patient population is a challenge for nurses."

Neutropenia

Neutropenia is a reduction in neutrophils, a type of white blood cell that helps fight infection. In oncology patients, common causes of neutropenia include chemotherapy, radiation therapy, immunotherapy, and bone-marrow transplant.[26] If a patient with neutropenia develops an infection, the infection can quickly result in the patient's death.[26]

Although many organizations promote the use of isolation precautions for immunocompromised patients, no evidence suggests that isolation reduces their risk of infection.[25] However, nurses should take care not to expose neutropenic patients to potentially infectious patients.[25] Visitors should also be screened for possible infections and instructed not to visit if symptoms of infection are present.[25]

In patients with neutropenia, the usual signs and symptoms of infection may not be present due to an insufficient number of neutrophils necessary to produce common signs of infection, such as pus or productive cough.[26] Nurses should monitor their oncology patients for the following signs and symptoms that may indicate infection[26]:

• Fever or chills
• Change in cough or new onset of cough

- Sore throat
- New mouth sore
- Burning or pain with urination
- Redness or swelling on any part of the body
- Pain at catheter site
- Diarrhea
- Abdominal or rectal pain
- Change in mental status

A temperature of 100.4°F (38°C) for greater than one hour or a single temperature of 101°F (38.3°C) in neutropenic patients requires that the medical team be informed. "In neutropenic patients, fever may be the only sign of infection," Zitella says.

Oral Mucositis

Oral mucositis is sores or ulcers that form on the lining of the inside of the mouth (mucous membranes) or on the lips.[27] It can be caused by chemotherapy or radiation of the head or neck.[27] Although no known methods for preventing oral mucositis exist, nurses should educate their oncology patients about things they can do to minimize their risk for developing mouth sores, such as the following[27]:

- **Go to the dentist before beginning chemotherapy or radiation treatments.** Any untreated pain or infections in the mouth will likely worsen after treatment.
- **Develop a mouth care routine.** This should include brushing the teeth and rinsing the mouth several times each day. It should also include flossing once a day. Avoid alcohol-based mouthwashes.
- **Stop smoking.** Smoking makes it more difficult for the mouth to heal itself.
- **Maintain a balanced diet.** Vitamins and nutrients from fruits and vegetables help the body fight infections.
- **Drink 2 to 3 quarts of water every day.** Staying hydrated enhances well-being and keeps the body running smoothly.

Patient Education

Oncology nurses play vital roles in educating patients and their families about infection prevention and control.[26] Patient education should include the following[26]:

- Wash hands frequently, especially after toileting and before eating.
- Avoid crowds and people with respiratory infections.
- Bathe daily.

- Perform routine mouth care as described above.
- Contact your doctor if you have signs and symptoms of infection.

Patients should be educated and treated according to research and national guidelines. "Sometimes, nursing advice is based on routine practice, culture, or opinion, rather than on evidence," Zitella says. "For example, patients are often advised to comply with a neutropenic diet, although research suggests that it does not reduce the risk of infection. Nurses should be familiar with the latest research and national guidelines and offer evidence-based advice when possible."

Case Example: Reducing Central Line-Associated Bloodstream Infections (CLABSIs)

A large children's hospital in the southwest United States recently began an initiative to try to decrease central line-associated bloodstream infection (CLABSI) rates in children with cancer.[28] The intervention was a comprehensive educational program aimed at staff nurses. The program included a didactic presentation, hands-on clinical simulation, and pre- and post-education assessment to evaluate learning.[28] The program focused on teaching strict adherence to aseptic technique, central line maintenance measures, and methods to reduce catheter hub colonization.[28]

The hospital monitored infection rates every month for six months after the program. Following implementation, infection rates reduced from 5.59 to 3.35 per 1,000 catheter-days for patients undergoing bone marrow transplantation and from 4.89 to 3.00 per 1,000 catheter-days for general cancer patients.[28]

Long Term Care

Residents of long term care facilities may be at risk for infection for many reasons. Most are elderly, and many have multiple comorbidities that may make it difficult to recognize symptoms of infection.[29] Additionally, most long term care facilities do not have equipment or personnel on site to evaluate patients with suspected infections as they would in acute care settings.[29]

One of the challenges that nurses face in preventing and controlling infection in long term care facilities is seeing that residents are given adequate assistance with hand hygiene. "Try to visualize a patient in a wheelchair," says Vicki Pritchard, surveyor, Long Term Care, The Joint Commission. "The resident is touching the wheel rim as it rolls across the floor, picking up who knows what kind of germs.

When the hands touch the nose, the mouth, or the eyes, the organisms get introduced into the system and cause infection. Nurses need to help residents with hand hygiene, particularly after toileting and before meals."

Urinary Tract Infections

UTIs are the most common type of HAI in long term care facilities. One of the difficulties with diagnosing UTIs in long term care facilities is that they are frequently asymptomatic.[29] In addition, when a resident does have symptoms, they may be atypical, so one of the major challenges for nurses is to determine which changes in a resident's condition may indicate the need for further evaluation and follow up by a physician.[29,30] Symptoms of UTIs in elderly patients may include the following[29-31]:

• Fever
• Chills
• Increased frequency of urination
• Flank pain
• Suprapubic tenderness
• New or increased incontinence
• Change in character of urine (color, odor)
• Decline in mental status accompanied by fever

Pneumonia

Pneumonia is the secondmost common type of HAI in long term care facilities.[31] As with UTIs, elderly patients with pneumonia may present with atypical symptoms, making it difficult for the nurse to determine when additional evaluation and follow-up are needed.[31] Symptoms may include the following[31]:

• Significant deterioration in ability to carry out activities of daily living
• Change in cognitive status
• Fever
• New or increased cough
• Respiratory rate greater than 25 breaths per minute

It has been suggested that, because elderly patients do present with atypical symptoms, the Minimum Data Set (MDS) and the Resident Assessment Instrument (RAI) be used to assess long term care residents for infection.[31] The MDS should be used to collect baseline data on admission and periodically thereafter. If changes are noted in mental status or ability to perform activities of daily living, the RAI can help identify infection.[31]

Equipment and Supplies

Medical equipment or supplies can be sources of infection in long term care residents. For example, in 2005, outbreaks of hepatitis B in two separate assisted living facilities in Virginia were traced to the sharing of routine glucose-monitoring equipment, including glucometers and spring-loaded fingerstick devices.[32] Because glucose-monitoring equipment comes into close proximity to blood every time it is used, the risk of infection from equipment sharing should be obvious.[32] To decrease the risk for infection, the Centers for Disease Control and Prevention (CDC) recommends that glucometers be assigned to individuals, if possible.[32] If not, they should be cleaned after each use.[32]

Another potential source for infection in long term care facilities is reprocessing of disposable items, such as bedpans or urinals. "Long term care employees will often collect all of the bedpans and urinals and soak them in one tub with disinfectant," Pritchard says. "Then they take them back and redistribute them, thinking they're clean, when they're really painted with filth. Some old nursing homes also have flushing systems where you stick the bedpan in, shut the door, and flush. Those systems are obsolete. These types of practices contribute to norovirus outbreaks or the spread of *C. diff.* Bedpans and urinals should be used for one patient only and should be emptied into the patient's toilet and rinsed using a spigot or spray. When they get old or begin to crack, they should be replaced." Bedpans and urinals should always be labeled with the patient's name to make it less likely for items to be used for the wrong patient.

The Long Term Care Challenge

One of the challenges to preventing and controlling infections in long term care facilities is the need to balance loving care with prevention of infection. "In long term care, there is a lot of hugging, touching, or close contact when moving patients," says Pritchard. "If a resident has an infection, focus on the mode of transmission, then determine how you can stop the spread of infection and still allow care to be as normalized as possible. For example, if a patient has a wound that is colonized with MRSA, if there is a secure dressing over the site and everyone is performing good hand hygiene, there is no need for isolation. So look at the resident, look at the mode of transmission, and see if there are measures you can take to control the spread of infection. If so, there's no need to isolate."

Case Example: Bradford Oaks Nursing and Rehabilitation Center, Clinton, Maryland

Bradford Oaks Nursing and Rehabilitation Center in Clinton, Maryland, set out to reduce the prevalence and incidence of UTIs as part of Delmarva Foundation's Nursing Home Quality Initiative.[33] It chose a pilot population that included all residents with a diagnosis of chronic bacteriuria and recurrent UTI. Its improvement program included the following six steps[33]:

1. A letter was sent to all attending physicians with a copy of the American Medical Directors Association (AMDA)/CDC guidelines for diagnosis and treatment of UTIs in the long term care setting.
2. An inservice was conducted for all licensed nurses.
3. Physician's orders were obtained for one cranberry 425 mg capsule twice a day for the pilot group.
4. Physician's orders were obtained for the use of silver-covered catheters for the pilot group.
5. A chart review was conducted to ensure that physicians were using the AMDA/CDC guidelines; a reminder letter was sent to physicians who were not using the guidelines.
6. An inservice was held for the MDS coordinator to ensure that quality indicators for UTIs were being coded correctly.

Over a three-year period, the prevalence of UTIs in the pilot group decreased from a monthly range of 5.6% to 9.2% to a monthly range of 0% to 1.5%.[33] The monthly incidence rates continue to hold steady at less than 1%. However, at one point, the rates did increase for two consecutive months but declined again after further staff education.[33]

Behavioral Health Care

The types of infections that are prevalent in behavioral health care are dependent upon the type of setting. According to Cynthia Leslie, A.P.R.N., M.S.N., associate director, Standards Interpretation Group, The Joint Commission, communicable diseases, such as measles, tuberculosis, influenza, scabies, lice, and MRSA, may be common to the inpatient setting. "When a patient is admitted to a facility, it is important to do a thorough assessment and obtain a complete history," Leslie says. "If the patient is a poor historian, it is important to obtain as much information as possible from the family or the patient's physician."

The introduction of an infectious disease into an inpatient facility can have a major impact on patient morbidity and mortality.[34] When an outbreak or a potential outbreak is detected, measures should be taken to prevent the spread of infection to other patients. These may include the implementation of contact precautions for symptomatic patients, good hand-hygiene practices, discouraging patients from leaving their rooms, cohorting of symptomatic patients, and instructing patients in performing hand hygiene and respiratory etiquette.[34,35]

The structure of inpatient behavioral health facilities poses challenges to infection prevention and control.[34] For example, patients in behavioral health facilities tend to live in rooms with two to four patients. They also share bathroom and shower facilities.[34] "In residential facilities, you get many clients from different walks of life," Leslie says. "They eat together, they watch television together. Since they are in such close proximity, they need to be taught what to do to prevent the spread of infection."

Patients with psychiatric illnesses create additional challenges due to their inability to sometimes comprehend instructions and a frequent failure to abide by activity restrictions.[34] Nurses can help prevent or control the spread of infection on psychiatric units by assisting patients with hand hygiene, cohorting symptomatic patients, and leading wandering patients away from communal areas.[34]

Outpatient Clinics

In outpatient behavioral health clinics, hepatitis C, HIV/AIDS, or other infections secondary to substance abuse are common.[36] Binge drinking and heavy drug use have been known to contribute to risky sexual behaviors, including trading sex for money, engaging in unprotected sex, and having numerous sexual partners.[36] People with psychiatric disorders may also have deficits in problem-solving skills and poor impulse control, which may cause them to engage in risky behaviors.[36]

Behavioral health nurses in the outpatient setting should routinely assess risk for HIV and other sexually transmitted diseases (STDs).[36] Questions to ask should include the following[36]:

• Frequency of vaginal, anal, and oral sex
• Number and gender of sexual partners
• HIV risk of sexual partners
• Whether the patient has traded sex for money or drugs
• Past and current symptoms of STDs
• Condom use

Nurses should also obtain a detailed history of substance abuse, particularly those drugs that are injected or inhaled, and inquire about sharing of needles.

Patient Population

Nurses in any type of setting need to know their patient population. "It is important for the organization to identify risks for the transmission and acquisition of infectious agents based on geographic location and community environment," Leslie says. "This should be incorporated into the organization's infection control plan."

Case Example: Managing an Influenza Outbreak on a Behavioral Health Unit

In January 2006, eight patients on a locked behavioral health unit began exhibiting flulike symptoms.[34] At the time, a total of 26 patients were on the unit. All had been ordered influenza immunizations the previous fall, but many had declined.[34] Staff members took the following steps to contain the outbreak[34]:

- Notified the infection preventionist and the hospital epidemiologist
- Instituted modified droplet precautions
- Conducted rapid antigen tests on symptomatic patients to identify the presence of influenza
- Closed the unit to admission and visitors
- Confined patients to the unit
- Transferred severely symptomatic patients to acute care, where they were placed on droplet precautions
- Cohorted the symptomatic patients that remained on the unit
- Encouraged the use of face masks
- Offered immunization and prophylaxis oseltamivir phosphate to asymptomatic patients
- Reinstructed patients in hand-hygiene techniques and respiratory etiquette
- Encouraged symptomatic employees to stay at home

Due to quick identification of the potential outbreak and steps taken to control the spread of infection, 18 of the 26 patients on the ward remained asymptomatic after the outbreak was identified. Only 8 out of 40 staff members became symptomatic.[34]

References

1. Sutter P., et al.: Telehealth infection control: A movement toward best practice. *Home Healthc Nurse* 27:319–323, May 2009.

2. Lord C.: Surgical-site infections after coronary artery bypass graft. *Home Healthc Nurse* 24:28–32, Jan. 2006.

3. Kenneley I.L.: Infection control and prevention in home healthcare: Prevention activities are the key to desired patient outcomes. *Home Healthc Nurse* 25:459–469, Jul.–Aug. 2007.

4. Thobaben M.: Centers for Disease Control and Prevention's (CDC) "An Ounce of Prevention—Keeps the Germs Away" Campaign. *Home Health Care Management and Practice* 20:498–500, Oct. 2008.

5. McGoldrick M.: Cleaning and disinfecting patient care equipment is an important infection prevention strategy for patients receiving care in the home. *Caring* pp. 34–39, Mar. 2009.

6. Gold K., Schumann J.: Dangers of used sharps in household trash: Implications for home care. *Home Healthc Nurse* 25:602–606, Oct. 2007.

7. U.S. Environmental Protection Agency: *Protect Yourself, Protect Others: Safe Options for Home Needle Disposal.* Oct. 2004. http://www.safeneedledisposal.org/assets/pdf/med-home.pdf (accessed Aug. 4, 2009).

8. Nurses' bags play key role in infection control. *Hospital Home Health* pp. 64–65, Jun. 2008.

9. American Academy of Pediatrics: Infection prevention and control in pediatric ambulatory settings. *Pediatrics* 120:650–665, Sep. 2007.

10. 4 steps that can improve infection control practices. *Same Day Surg* pp. 55–58, May 2008.

11. Allen G.: Targeting zero: Preventing infections in ambulatory settings. *AORN* 88:891–892, May 2008.

12. *Surgery Programs Reduce Infections to Zero, or Close.* http://www.spiveystationsurgerycenter.com/f/6.1.09_Same-Day_Surgery_Surgery_programs_reduce_infections_to_zero_or_close.pdf (accessed Aug. 13, 2009).

13. How to get staff to wash their hands. *Same Day Surg* p. 57, Jun. 2009.

14. 3 ways you can stop infections in your ED. *ED Nursing* pp. 123–124, Sep. 2008.

15. EDs not taking chances with H1N1, protocols updated, supplies checked. *ED Manag* 21:61–63, Jun. 2009.

16. Is infection "present on admission" in your ED? *ED Nursing* pp.77–78, May 2009.

17. Tepus D., et al.: Effectiveness of Chloraprep™ in reduction of blood culture contamination rates in emergency department. *J Nurs Care Qual* 23:272–276, Jul.–Sep. 2008.

18. Tom-Revzon C.: Strategic use of antibiotics in the neonatal intensive care unit. *J Perinat Neonatal Nurs* 18:241–258, Jul.–Sep. 2004.

19. Barford G., Rentz A.C., Faix R.G.: Viral infection and antiviral therapy in the neonatal intensive care unit. *J Perinat Neonatal Nurs* 18:259–274, Jul.–Sep. 2004.

20. Murillo J.L.: *Newborn MRSA Surveillance Questionnaire.* Newark, NJ: Newark Beth Israel Medical Center, 2008.

21. Norris S.C., Barnes A.K., Roberts T.D.: When ventilator-associated pneumonias haunt your ICU—One unit's story. *Neonatal Netw* 28:59–66, Jan.–Feb. 2009.

22. Rose P., Blythe S.: Use of single rooms on the children's ward: Part 1. *Paediatr Nurs* 20:13–17, Dec. 2008.

23. Fleming K., Randle J.: Toys—Friend or foe? A study of infection risk in a paediatric intensive care unit. *Paediatr Nurs* 18:14–18, May 2006.

24. Chen Y.C., Chiang L.C.: Effectiveness of hand-washing teaching programs for families of children in paediatric intensive care units. *J Clin Nurs* 16:1173–1179, Jun. 2007.

25. Zitella L.J., et al.: Putting evidence into practice: Prevention of infection. *Clin J Oncol Nurs* 10:739–750, Dec. 2006.

26. Marrs J.A.: Care of patients with neutropenia. *Clin J Oncol Nurs* 10:164–166, Apr. 2006.

27. Mayo Foundation for Medical Education and Research: *Mouth Sores: Cancer-Related Causes and How to Cope.* http://www.mayoclinic.com/health/mouth-sores/CA00054 (accessed Aug. 10, 2009).

28. Horvath B., et al.: Reducing central venous catheter-related bloodstream infections in children with cancer. *Oncol Nurs Forum* 36:232–238, Mar. 2009.

29. High K.P., et al.: Clinical practice guideline for the evaluation of fever and infection in older adult residents of long-term care facilities: 2008 update by the Infectious Diseases Society of America. *J Am Geriatr Soc* 57:375–394, Mar. 2009.

30. Midthum S.J.: Criteria for urinary tract infection in the elderly: Variables that challenge nursing assessment. *Urol Nurs* 24:157–170, Jun. 2004.

31. Goldrick B.A.: Infection in the older adult. *Am J Nurs* 105:31–34, Jun. 2005.

32. Patel A.S., et al.: Infection control practices in assisted living facilities: A response to hepatitis B virus infection outbreaks. *Infect Control Hosp Epidemiol* 30:209–214, Mar. 2009.

33. McMullen D., Bartlett J.M., Rosario J.G.: *A Long-Term Care Facility Attacks UTI Prevalence: Implementing a Team Approach to Increase Staff Knowledge of and Compliance with Good Infection Control Practices.* May 1, 2007. http://www.allbusiness.com/health-care-social-assistance/nursing/4505334-1.html (accessed Aug. 13, 2009).

34. Risa K.J., McAndrew J.M., Muder R.R.: Influenza outbreak management on a locked behavioral health unit. *Am J Infect Control* 37:76–78, Feb. 2009.

35. Gillbride S.J., et al.: Successful containment of a norovirus outbreak in an acute adult psychiatric area. *Infect Control Hosp Epidemiol* 30:289–291, Mar. 2009.

36. Dyer J.G., McGuinness T.M.: Reducing HIV risk among people with serious mental illness. *J Psychosoc Nurs Ment Health Serv* 46:26–34, Apr. 2008.

Index